COMMON SENSE ABOUT DYSLEXIA

By

Anne Marshall Huston

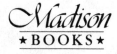

★ BOOKS ★

LANHAM • NEW YORK • LONDON

Library of Congress Cataloging in Publication Data

Huston, Anne Marshall.
    Common sense about dyslexia.

    Bibliography: p.
    Includes index.
    1. Dyslexia—Popular works.   I. Title. [DNLM:
1. Dyslexia—Popular works.   WL   340.6   H842c]
RC394.W6H87   1986   616.85'53   86-23689
ISBN 0-8191-6323-6 (alk. paper)
ISBN 0-8191-5666-3 (pbk. : alk. paper)

All Madison Books are produced on acid-free
paper which exceeds the minimum standards set by the National
Historical Publications and Records Commission.

★ BOOKS ★

To
JIM
sine qua non

TABLE OF CONTENTS

PART TWO: THE LANGUAGE DISCONNECTION, DYSLEXIA

Chapter 3 25
Overview of the Common Characteristics of Dyslexic Students

Chapter 4 41
Visual Dyslexia

Chapter 15

What Can Teachers Do?

PREFACE

This book is a response in part to many requests from parents, teachers, reading and learning disability specialists, other school personnel involved with students who have special problems, physicians, and, yes, children who have dyslexia. It is the result of over fifteen years of study, research, and experience with dyslexia in public schools, college classrooms, graduate programs, and a reading clinic for the diagnosis and remediation of reading disabilities and dyslexia, which actually is a disability in writing, spelling, speaking, and listening, as well as reading.

Dyslexia is a language communication disability. It includes three general categories. The first, visual dyslexia, is characterized by reversals of letters and numerals; faulty sequencing of letters in words, numbers in series, and events in narrative; disorientation in time and space relationships; and problems in processing, interpreting, and recalling visual images. The second, auditory dyslexia, is characterized by problems of integrating and processing what is heard and recalling those sounds and applying them to the printed symbols representing them. The third is a combination of the two in varying degrees. Dyslexia is not attributable to any vision or hearing defect; it persists beyond that time when most childhood developmental conditions mature.

The prefix "dys" (Greek) means defective, as in dysfunction; that is, a functional abnormality or impairment—and "lexia" (Greek) refers to the use of words.

Words are the means by which we communicate in our language. And dyslexia is certainly a problem with words—in reading, spelling, writing, speaking, and listening. Unfortunately, in the past some have confused dyslexia with the Latin "lexit" (having to do with reading, or "he has read"). Although, in consequence, in some of the textbooks dyslexia can be found to be inappropriately defined as a "general term meaning inability to read" or "a reading disorder," dyslexia is *much more than just a reading disability.* Dyslexia is a *language communication disability.*

Disagreement over the "right" definition creates much dissatisfaction and is sometimes cited to support the contention that dyslexia must not exist if the experts cannot agree on a common definition. Yet pick up a dozen textbooks on how to teach reading and you are likely to find a dozen different definitions of "reading."

We need to keep our feet on the ground when considering dyslexia. We need to use our common sense. We must cut through the controversies in the academic and medical worlds about what particular definition to use, what causes dyslexia, or whether it exists at all. There are authorities in medicine, psychology, learning disabilities, and reading who acknowledge the existence of dyslexia, while others (mainly in the reading field) deny its existence as a distinct affliction or condition. What is needed at this time is better communication and cooperation which will, of course, result in better understanding. The important thing to keep in mind is that *the focus must always be on the children and their problems.*

There is something of a hue and cry going on about "labeling" children with the term "dyslexia." Several reading "authorities" prefer the term "severe reading disability"—as if that were not just another label (and at that probably more frightening considering the use of the word "severe"). Special education authorities will place dyslexic children in "learning disabilities" classes—again, just another label. Why do we go on and on about it? Such terms as word-blindness, strephosymbolia, primary reading disability, secondary reading disability, constitutional reading disability, developmental dyslexia, specific dyslexia, maturational dyslexia, specific language disability, and others have been used. Each becomes a "label," and so we move on to try another term, which then becomes another label . . .

In the Library of Congress there are over 170 books about dyslexia, published in sixteen countries. There are 2,394 entries in Evans' *Dyslexia, An Annotated Bibliography,* including journal articles, conference reports, proceedings of symposia, government documents, chapters or parts of books, dissertations, and articles from the popular press. Articles about dyslexia have appeared in *Medical Science, Journal of Genetic Psychology, Annals of Neurology, Developmental Medicine and Child Neurology, Journal of the American Medical Association, Lancet, British Journal of Educational Psychology, Learning Disabilities,* and journals published by the International Reading Association.

While there have been many books, articles, and studies about dyslexia over the years, programs and methods suggested in many of them are now outdated as a result of our continuing growth in knowledge and experience with dyslexia. Some books recommend a "cookbook" approach to remediation, often with commercial emphasis on buying a particular program—on the assumption that the child needs everything, so give him the whole program. They do not take into account what he already knows, nor what he specifically needs. Some authors tend to sit on the fence and try to be all things to all persons, never taking a stand, with a "Well, this might work or that might work." Still other books are comprehensive reviews of the literature on dyslexia which present series after series of studies, one contradicting the other, with very few firm conclusions. Don't misunderstand. There *is* a need for professional comprehensive surveys of the literature on dyslexia. But one must always read the studies with a critical eye. The validity of any research study should be questioned on the basis of its sampling procedures, the use or lack of control groups, the size of the population tested, the accuracy of the diagnosis of "alleged" dyslexia, the length of time of treatment, information about actual hours of teaching, the training of the teachers, the percentage of children who remain available for post-testing, and so on. A further important consideration ignored in most studies is the subtypes of dyslexia. Lumping all dyslexics together tends to make the subtypes neutralize the data in many ways. A difference in numbers in the subtypes, if grouped together in one study, could result in a skewing of certain results.

This book represents the first of two volumes on dyslexia. It has been written for parents of dyslexics, classroom teachers, and principals, and for those who are interested in learning more about this challenging problem. This book is not intended to be used for diagnostic purposes. The second volume will deal with the actual diagnosis and remediation of dyslexia and will be directed at those charged with this responsibility in our schools—the reading specialists and learning disability teachers—who have had professional training at the graduate levels in the language arts areas and in testing and remediation.

This is intended as a practical book to help understand dyslexia. Every effort has been made to keep it readable and to avoid the typical educational jargon that can be so confusing to parents and even the classroom teacher. Certain special terms have been explained when necessary. A glossary is provided at the end of the book.

We are excited about what is happening to our understanding of dyslexia. The more children we can help—both at the clinic and after they return to their schools and classrooms and through those who read this book—the more worthwhile and contented citizens we will have. And all those years of work and study and trying this and that to find what works best, and caring and agonizing with each student who has passed through our doors—will have been worth it all.

Common sense is not so common.
—*Voltaire*

ACKNOWLEDGEMENTS

In addition to the specific acknowledgements that have been made in appropriate chapters in this book, I wish to thank the following for their help and for all that I have learned from them over the years:

— all those boys and girls who have come to me seeking help for their various problems,

—and their parents who have shared their concerns and heartache so candidly,

—and the children's teachers who worked so hard to help their students but knew additional help was needed, and who were so willing to share information and so appreciative of our work with their students,

—my highly dedicated graduate students who spent many conscientious hours planning and preparing not only the work required for our classes but also for those children whose strengths and difficulties had to be uncovered and the latter remediated insofar as was possible. These knowledge-seeking, caring students have been a continuing source of inspiration to me,

—Mrs. Mary Scudder, Mrs. Marjorie Freeman, Mrs. Carol Pollock, Mrs. Deborah Beckel, Mrs. Helen Bryant, and all the personnel at the Lynchburg College Library for they were always graciously willing to help find certain books and journals, obtain books and copies of articles through interlibrary loan, and help make my research easier any way they could,

—Dr. Julius Sigler and Dr. James Carico who took time from their busy schedules to sit down with me and introduce me to the use of the word processor—and the spelling program,

—those at the College Computer Lab for they, too, were always ready and willing to give me help whenever I needed it. Special thanks go to Kipp Teague and Gail Troy, and to Greg Bailey, Chris Johnson, Paul Johnson, Bryan Justice, and Partha Lahiri,

—Dr. Orrie O. Stenroos for his help in obtaining research on twin placentation,

—Mrs. Phyllis Lane and her skillful typing of the appendices, glossary, and bibliography,

—the mother, who cannot be named, who gave me permission to reproduce her letter concerning the problems her son had been having in school,

—the five children described in Chapter Seven and whose names have been changed to assure confidentiality,

—Lynchburg College for providing me with a year's sabbatical leave so that I might complete this book, and to my husband, Jim, who was always there to give me help, encouragement, and inspiration through the long hours of researching and organizing information, writing and rewriting and proofreading.

A.M.H.

PART ONE: GETTING A PERSPECTIVE

We have endeavored . . . to observe a kind of perspective, that one part may cast light upon another.
—*Francis Bacon*

CHAPTER
1

INTRODUCTION TO THE DYSLEXIA PROBLEM

Yet all experience is an arch
wherethrough gleams that untraveled world.

—*Tennyson*

My office telephone rang late one October afternoon, and when I answered I heard a woman's voice. She was obviously very agitated. "My daughter has dyslexia! What can I do?"

"Your child has dyslexia?" I asked. "How do you know she has dyslexia?" This is a question that I have learned always to ask.

"Because my sister says so," came back the reply.

"Your *sister*? Who is she? How did she come to this conclusion?" This is another question I have learned always to ask.

"She was at the beauty salon and she read an article in one of those parents' magazines that said if a child reverses *b* and *d* or *p* and *q* then the child is probably dyslexic. What are we to do? Can you help us?"

"Now hold on a minute," I answered. "I need more information than that."

I asked her what grade her daughter was in, thinking that if she were in the third or fourth grade (or higher), there *might* be problems of some kind. But the child was in the first grade. I asked her age and was told that she was not yet six years old. I inquired as to the date of her birth and was told that she was born in December. This made her a "young first-grader." (Unfortunately, in our state at that time, children could enter first grade in September if they had their sixth birthday before the following January 1, a ruling that disturbed many professional early childhood educators.)

I explained to the mother that it is normal for a child of that age to re-verse those letters. I asked if she had had her daughter's vision checked, since certain types of visual defects can cause these difficulties. She had. I explained that the reversal problems would probably disappear by the end of the second grade, or perhaps even earlier. I also asked her to keep in touch with me and to let me know if the difficulty continued beyond that time.

It did not. By the end of the second grade the child was reading and writ-ing without reversals of any kind. When I followed up, the mother recalled how upset and frightened she had been. "How could I have been so foolish?" she asked. "If only I had used some common sense instead of going off on a tangent. I should have known better!"

This child did not have dyslexia, but the story is a good example of how parents and educators can be thrown off the track by "popular" articles written by persons who do not have the training and experience to diagnose dyslexia, nor an understanding of child growth and development and how these are re-lated to the reading/spelling/writing processes. Such misinformation is not limited to popular articles. My telephone nearly rang off the hook after a speech by an educational psychologist at our local learning disabilities meet-ing at which he informed the audience that "any child who, at age five, reverses *b* and *d*, *p* and *q*, *saw* and *was*, *no* and *on*, *tap* and *pat*, is a dyslexic." Unfor-tunately, the local newspaper picked this up, and the statement appeared in the next morning's paper, frightening many parents unnecessarily. How many five year olds are reading those words anyhow? And if they *are*, they are prob-ably not dyslexic.

Scare tactics have no place where children and parents are concerned. Nor where educators are concerned. "Diagnosing off the top of the head" not only adds fuel to the dyslexia credibility controversy, it contributes to the mis-diagnosis of children and the creation of new problems, and to needless anx-iety on the part of parents.

When the Child has Dyslexia

It may be something of a relief when the diagnosis indicates that the child is not a dyslexic, but can be classified as a remedial reader or a corrective reader—neither of which is as serious as dyslexia and therefore can be more easily and quickly alleviated. But at times this is not the case. The evidence is there and common sense tells us that a spade must be called a spade. When this is done the door is open for remediating the dyslexic difficulties. For the child with dyslexia *can* be helped. Success in alleviating dyslexia is one of the most encouraging developments in education in recent years.

Dyslexia, What is It?

The word "dyslexia" has been bandied about, passed back and forth, been the subject of dissension among friends, left many in a quandary, or in disbelief, and so much so that if it could speak it would tell us that it is as bruised as the undiagnosed dyslexic child himself.

Dyslexia is more than just a reading disability. The word itself refers to a dysfunction or impairment in the use of words. The Greek prefix "dys" means defective, as in dysfunction; that is, a functional abnormality or impairment. The Greek "lexia" refers to the use of words (not just reading). And words are the means of communication in language—in reading, yes, but also in writing, in speaking, and in listening. Words are used in all school subjects, whether it be math or science or social studies or any other. Students listen for instruction, read the textbooks for information, write reports or other papers, copy work from the chalkboard or overhead projector, or solve mathematical problems (thinking as they work, for example, that "six plus four equals ten"— in *words*).

The dyslexic may not only confuse letters in reading and writing such as *m* with *w*, *n* with *u*, *b* with *d*, or *p* with *q*, but may confuse numerals in math and science, such as *2* with *5* or *6* with *9*. Problems in sequencing, such as getting letters out of order within words, will cause a dyslexic to switch the order of digits in numbers, such as 245 for 254 or 1856 for 1865. This applies to dates in history as well as numbers in math and science. It is also likely to lead to the transposition of notes when reading music. Sequencing problems contribute confusion in a variety of ways: with the occurrence of events in a basal reader story or in social studes with events that have happened in history, or the use of the time line; as well as with the sequential steps in a science experiment, or in math when working long division or word problems; and with following directions, whether written or spoken, in any subject.

Dyslexia is a language communication disability. It includes three general categories. The first, visual dyslexia, is characterized by reversals of letters and numerals; faulty sequencing of letters in words, numbers in series, and events in narrative; disorientation in time and space relationships; and problems in processing, interpreting, and recalling visual images. The second, auditory dyslexia, is characterized by problems of integrating and processing what is heard and recalling those sounds and applying them to the printed symbols representing them. The third is a combination of the two in varying degrees. Dyslexia is not attributable to any vision or hearing defect; it persists beyond that time when most childhood developmental conditions normally mature.

Dyslexia consists of a syndrome of characteristics which varies in degree according to the severity and kind of dyslexia in the individual. Just as one can have the symptoms of a mild or a severe chest cold, so, too, with dyslexia. And just as a severe chest cold can go into pneumonia if not treated, so, too, the child with severe dyslexia can become a failure in life, a dropout in our society.

Dyslexia, Who has It?

The Incidence of Dyslexia

There is no general agreement about the total number of dyslexics in our population. Estimates range from 2 percent to 25 percent, depending upon the study or source. The terminology itself can be confusing and misleading. In books and reviews on dyslexia, the subjects of studies are referred to in various ways, such as being "learning disabled," "reading retarded," "reading disabled," having "specific learning difficulties," or being "dyslexic." The results of these studies are often compared with one another. And the results of studies on substantially normal populations have been applied indiscriminately to dyslexics—a most questionable procedure. Moreover, since studies done on dyslexics have not, in most cases, differentiated among the categories of dyslexia, the results will certainly confound the findings. All this brings the validity of a great deal of the research on dyslexia into question.

The accuracy of the diagnoses of dyslexia must also be considered. Were the subjects used in a particular study actually dyslexic? For example, some researchers use as the criterion for determining dyslexia simply as reading two or more grades below grade placement on the basis of standardized reading achievement tests. This is wrong. And literal interpretation of the grade equivalent scores of the standardized tests should be avoided. There are various measurement and interpretive problems with such procedures that can affect any conclusions.[1]

Some children who read below grade level are simply slow learners; they are not necessarily dyslexic. They are intellectually unable to read at a particular grade level. A student may have been ill, had to take time out from school, and thus gotten behind in his reading achievement. Perhaps emotional trauma, such as the death of a parent, interfered with a child's learning progress in school, or with his performance during testing. Again a child may have changed schools and fallen behind because what he had yet to learn had already been covered in his new classroom. There are many reasons why students can be performing two grades below grade level, *other than being dyslexic*. In short, a child may be a "remedial reader" but not a dyslexic. Far too many studies have not taken this into account.

A study cited in a "current" book compared 7- and 8-year-old normal boys with dyslexic boys of the same age and found that the normal group was better able to recognize melody patterns in oral language. In this study a child was labeled *dyslexic* if he was reading below grade level and had average intelligence.[2] Incredible! *Any* child reading below grade level and of average intelligence being called dyslexic! No wonder there are skeptics. No wonder there is a credibility gap.

There are also children who have been misdiagnosed by poorly trained specialists on the basis of only a few characteristics symptomatic of dyslexia. Diagnoses have been made solely on a student's spelling errors rather than on the results of a battery of tests with consideration of the child's performance in various areas in order to obtain a comprehensive diagnostic perspective of his overall strengths and weaknesses. An excellent reader may be a poor speller. Indeed, a teacher's method of teaching spelling and reading can affect a child's accuracy and create certain patterns of spelling or reading errors. At times, incorrect diagnoses of dyslexia have occurred when attempting to make a decision of dyslexia in a child who is too young. If these children are used as part of the population in comparative studies, obviously the findings will not be valid. On the other hand, if those children in our schools who do have dyslexia, but are so far undiagnosed, were used in the control groups of studies, the waters would be muddied even more.

Here are examples of two extreme viewpoints about the incidence of dyslexia in schools: One principal of an elementary school has said that there "are no dyslexic children in my school." Yet four dyslexic boys attend his school. Since they are not getting the help they need at school, the parents have had to employ a reading specialist, trained in remediating dyslexia, to work with the boys on a private basis after school. Admittedly, dyslexic students can be a real bother to the administrator. They also tend to lower that "all-important" standardized test average on which schools appear to place so much significance. (Yet if the dyslexics were helped, it would raise that average.)

The principal of another elementary school in the same system told me that she has "a whole school full of dyslexics." Since both schools are "typical" elementary schools with similar populations, it is not likely that one of them, with some hundreds of children, would have no dyslexics, and that the other would be "full of dyslexics."

The incidence of dyslexia? Common sense, experience, and the reasons stated above suggest that a range of from 2 percent to 5 percent is probably a plausible estimate of the incidence of dyslexia. The incidence of *reading retardation* in the schools may be as high as 25 percent, *but not that of dyslexia.*

Dyslexia Around the World

Dyslexia is not limited to any one country or region of the world. In the Library of Congress there are books about dyslexia which have been published in Australia, Austria, Belgium, Canada, Czechoslovakia, Chile, Denmark, France, Germany, Great Britain, Hungary, Holland, the Philippines, and Portugal, as well as the United States. There have been International World

Congresses on Dyslexia. Numerous articles have been written in various medical and other professional journals over a period of many years. The incidence of dyslexia as reported varies a great deal from language to language, with the lowest reported for Japanese and the highest usually for English.[3] There has been much speculation as to the reason. One assumption is that the answer may lie in the inherent linguistic merits and script of the different languages. However, Critchley—and others—maintains that this is not credible and suggests the more likely explanation that in Japan the neurologists, educational psychologists, and teachers are not so sensitive to the occurrence of dyslexia. If this were to prove wrong, then Critchley suggests the low incidence of dyslexia in Japan might be due to genetic reasons.[4] At any rate, at the present time, this variance of dyslexia from language to language cannot be explained. What we *do* know is that dyslexia is likely to be found around the world.

Are there Sex Differences?

There are sex differences in the incidence of dyslexia just as there are in color blindness. The dyslexic child is referred to in most books as "he" for a good reason. While both boys and girls can have dyslexia, boys are far more likely to have it.

As with estimates on the incidence of dyslexia, so too, there is a lack of consensus on the ratio of dyslexic males to dyslexic females. The estimates vary from study to study: 2-to-1,[5] 3.5-to-1 or 4-to-1,[6] 4-to-1,[7] 5-to-1.[8] In our clinic the ratio of dyslexic males to dyslexic females has been 6.7-to-1.

The difference in the number of male dyslexics as compared to females is well-founded and accepted. The *reason* has not yet been established, although there are numerous hypotheses: a greater occurrence of cerebral trauma in males, the hemispheric functioning of the sexes, a mutant at a single locus whose expression is modified by sex, or a polygenic expression that has a lower threshold for males than for females.

What about Intelligence?

Perhaps because of the wording in some of the definitions of dyslexia and learning disabilities in articles and books about dyslexia, the erroneous idea has arisen that dyslexics must be average or above average in intelligence. This misconception may be partly due to well-meaning teachers who are sensitive to the needs of parents to know that their child does not lack intelligence, and of the child who may fear that he really is "a dummy" since he has so much trouble doing school work and cannot keep up with his classmates. To encourage parents and children, teachers will mention the names of famous people said to have had dyslexia—Einstein, for instance. (Actually, the evidence that Einstein was dyslexic is very weak. More is said about this in Chapter Twelve, "Some Notable People, Dyslexic or Not?")

Slow learners, average learners, superior learners—any can have dyslexia. The odds are that the child is likely to be of average or above average intelligence simply because about 75 percent of the population falls in those categories (50 percent average, 25 percent above the average range). But the slow learner can also have dyslexia, in which case diagnosis may be more difficult, and remediation will take longer.

Socioeconomic Background

Dyslexia has no favorites in regard to the wealthy or the poor, the cultured or the culturally disadvantaged. Any child from any background can have dyslexia. Money *can* be useful to the dyslexic child from the standpoint of getting private diagnostic help and private tutoring when the schools do not provide adequate services, but the socioeconomic backgrounds of dyslexics are varied.

Birth Order of Dyslexics

Any child in the family can have dyslexia, whether he be the oldest, the youngest, or the in-between child. Research on birth order is sparse. In a study of five hundred dyslexics, 24.6 percent were the oldest in their families while 36 percent were the youngest.[9] In another study no differences in birth order in the incidence of dyslexia among brothers and sisters were found in 112 families with dyslexics.[10] And in yet another study of 125 children (one hundred boys, twenty-five girls), the birth order of those with alleged dyslexia were as follows:

	Males	Females
First born	31	6
Second born	39	9
Third born	20	5
Fourth born	5	5
Fifth born	3	-
Adopted	2	-

Of those listed above as first born, nine were actually the only child in a family.[11]

In a study of fifty-four dyslexic students, I found fifteen to be first born, twenty to be second born, thirteen to be third born, and six to be fourth born. Of those first born, six were the only child in the family.

Summary

Dyslexia is a language communication disability, affecting reading, writing, speaking, and listening. It is a dysfunction or impairment in the use of words. Consequently, relations with others and performance in every subject in school can be affected by dyslexia. It can be found around the world, principally among boys. It exists in learners of slow, average, and superior intelligence. The dyslexic child can come from any background, or any income level; and dyslexia may occur in any child in a family regardless of the order in which he is born.

Notes for Chapter 1

1. Summarized in Wayne Otto and Richard J. Smith, *Corrective and Remedial Teaching* (Boston: Houghton Mifflin, 1980), p. 196.

2. In the upper grades, the grade equivalent scores do not represent the extent of contrast between raw score medians (for grades immediately above and below) that are indicated by grade equivalents in lower grades. A grade equivalent of one year below a child's grade placement in the second grade would thus signify a larger deviation from the raw score average for the second grade than would a grade equivalent score which is one year below placement in an upper grade. In addition, there is an inclination for grade equivalents to exaggerate minor differences between scores as a result of the curve fitting operations, and, therefore, large variations within groups tend to be indistinct. A student who is only a little above or below the median for his grade on a particular reading achievement test might seem to be much farther away from this criterion. Another problem with using the grade placement criteria is that some achievement tests use different forms at the different grade levels. Frank R. Vellutino, *Dyslexia: Theory and Research* (Cambridge, Mass.: MIT Press, 1980), p. 26.

3. P. G. Aaron, "The Neuropsychology of Developmental Dyslexia," *Reading Disorders, Varieties and Treatments,* R. N. Malatesha and P. G. Aaron, eds. (New York: Academic Press, 1982), p. 53.

4. Macdonald Critchley, *The Dyslexic Child* (Springfield, Illinois: Charles C. Thomas, 1970), p. 96.

5. John Money, "Dyslexia: A Postconference Review," *Reading Disability, Progress and Research Needs in Dyslexia,* John Money, ed. (Baltimore: Johns Hopkins, 1962), p. 31.

6. T. R. Miles and Elaine Miles, *Help for Dyslexic Children* (London: Methuen, 1983), p. 2.

7. Critchley, op.cit., p. 91.

8. Sandhya Naidoo, *Specific Dyslexia, The Research Report of the ICAA Word Blind Centre for Dyslexia Children* (New York: John Wiley & Sons, 1972), p. 25.

9. Edith Klasen, *The Syndrome of Specific Dyslexia* (Baltimore: University Park, 1972), p. 160.

10. Bertil Hallgren, *Specific Dyslexia ("Congenital Word-Blindness"); A Clinical and Genetic Study* (Copenhagen: Ejnar Munksgaard, 1950); trans. by Erica Odelberg (Stockholm: Esselte aktiebolag, 1950), p. 192.

11. Critchley, op.cit., p. 92.

CHAPTER

2

THE LANGUAGE CONNECTION: READING, WRITING, SPEAKING, LISTENING

Through experience and through language we learn.
Experience needs language to give it form. Language needs
experience to give it content.

—*Walter Loban*

Thought is not merely expressed in words; it comes into
existence through them.

—*Vygotsky*

Understanding Our Language

Since dyslexia is a language communication disability, we must understand our language and what is involved in reading, writing, speaking, and listening before we can understand dyslexia.

Language is the medium of communication. Human beings communicate their ideas and feelings through language—writing and reading, speaking and listening. Writing and speaking are called *expressive* language processes because information emerges from us in the form of spoken or written words to be heard or read by others. Reading and listening are called *receptive* language processes because that which is read and heard filters into us for processing. We receive information from the author or the speaker. Oral reading is a function of both expressive and receptive language.

We communicate through the words of our language. Words involve a reciprocal relationship—we not only express our thoughts in words, but our ideas come into being through them. Our thoughts are a form of inner speech.

While there are about 2,800 languages spoken in the world today,[1] we are interested here in our own language, English, although many words from other languages have crept into our vocabulary. Our young people often prefer *pizza* or *lasagna* to *broccoli* (Italian). Some like *sauerkraut* (German). They may prefer to *ski* rather than to hear a *saga* (Scandinavian), or to *skate* or sail on a *yacht* (Dutch). Others like to slap on a *sombrero*, sit on the *patio*, and play their *guitar* (Spanish). Young girls may like a touch of *rouge* (French) before going to the *bazaar* (Persian) for a cup of *coffee* (Turkish) on the *Sabbath* (Hebrew).

Our language is flexible, adaptable, and ever changing. In addition to adopting numerous words from other languages, we are continually coining new words and incorporating them into American English. The advent of the computer or any other discovery has created additional words which are now a part of our language. Indeed, other countries are now adopting our new American words (weekend, car, drugstore, stop).

The words in our language represent ideas or objects; that is, they are symbolic, but of course this is arbitrary and may change with time. Many words have changed in meaning since their inception. For some words, today's definition is not anything at all like the original meaning. For example, in Shakespeare's day *let* meant the same as *stop* does today—that is, it held the opposite meaning. And Shakespeare used the word *owe* as we now would use the word *own*.[2] Often young people and adults enjoy browsing through books dealing with word origins and the remarkable ways that some of our words have come into the language—Merriam's *Picturesque Word Origins* for young students, or Mencken's *The American Language*, or A. L. Rowse's introductions to his Contemporary Shakespeare Series, "Why a Contemporary Shakespeare?"[3]

Our language tends to be quite orderly with patterns of expressions that help us to anticipate what is coming next, whether we are listening or reading. Language is thus systematic with common elements which enable us to understand one another. There is a kind of information processing that occurs when we get meaning from an acoustic signal while we are listening to a speaker or from a printed text while we are reading.[4] And it is with this information processing that the dyslexic has difficulty.

Applying Sound to Symbol

Certain irregularities in our language make reading and writing especially difficult for dyslexics. This also applies to those students who have been limited to a phonics approach to reading or have had an overemphasis of the phonics word recognition strategy. These words may pose no problem in our everyday speaking and listening. It is when we see them in a book or try to write them, confusion often occurs. Pronounce aloud to yourself the following series of words; listen to what you are saying; and notice the similarity in spelling and the inconsistency in how they sound.

do/go	does/goes/shoes	fat/father
gave/have	hour/four/tour	man/many
alive/give	but/put; but/buy	key/they
on/one	her/here/there	brown/grown
small/shall	ought/bough/cough	home/some
catch/watch	bead/bread/break	ash/wash

Venezky[5] suggests that, in order to be more precise, words such as the above should be referred to as being *predictable* or *unpredictable*, rather than *regular* or *irregular* as is usually done because of the variance of pronunciation of the phonic elements even though they are written alike. At any rate, since the dyslexic's perception of even predictable words tends to be unstable and insecure, the irregular or unpredictable words present greater and more frustrating obstacles.

Irregular (or unpredictable) words, which are basically "exceptions to the phonics rules," must be incorporated into a child's sight vocabulary so that he can recognize them instantly without having to resort to various strategies to figure them out. Such words give visual dyslexics a great deal of trouble because they must rely on visual recall for these irregularities. The auditory dyslexic can draw more on visual recall, but, he too, has trouble because of all the sound variations, "silent" letters, and so forth.

In our spoken language we have various words which we understand when we *hear* them, but when this language is transferred to print or needs to be written, complications arise. Words that sound alike but have different meanings and spellings (called homophones or homonyms) such as *meet/meat, blew/blue,* or *pair/pear/pare* confuse the dyslexic. Then we also have words that are spelled alike but have different meanings and different pronunciations (called homographs) such as *produce* (pró duce), as the vegetables in your garden, and *produce* (pro ducé), as in the sentence, "Hens produce eggs." And we have words like *read* which can occur in this manner,

"I will read that book which you read last week." (The latter *read* sounds like the color *red*.) And so on.

The following poem cleverly but accurately illustrates the inconsistencies in the relationship of spoken language and written language:

Our Queer Language

When the English Tongue we speak
Why is "break" not rhymed with "freak"?
Will you tell me why it's true
We say "sew" and likewise "few"?
And the maker of the verse
Cannot cap his "horse" with "worse"?
"Beard" sounds not the same as "heard"
"Cord" is different from "word"
Cow is "cow" but low is "low"
"Shoe" is never rhymed with "foe"
Think of "hose" and "dose" and "lose"
And think of "goose" and not of "choose"
"Doll" and "roll," "home" and "some"
And since "pay" is rhymed with "say"
Why not "paid" with "said" I pray?
"Mould" is not pronounced like "could"
Where "done" but "gone" and "lone"
Is there any reason known?
And in short it seems to me
Sounds and letters disagree.

—Anon.

A bit confusing, isn't it? But, while our language appears rather complicated, and the connection seems to break down somewhat when we try to match it in print, most people *do* master the interrelationships of our language. The important point is that one must always be thinking, be understanding what is being said and what is being read.

This emphasis on meaning is critical for the dyslexic and is the connecting thread that matches oral language to a written language; that is, the sounds of words matched to the symbols that represent them on paper. Thinking, understanding, making associations, form the strongest means that a dyslexic can have to help him progress.

Understanding Reading

Reading is a form of communication by language. The author is trying to convey his thoughts to the reader through the medium of print. There is seldom, if ever, a perfect match of thought between the reader and the author. While the author knows what is in his own mind, the reader cannot "see" into the author's mind. He sees only the printed words on the page. There is no meaning *per se* in those printed words. Images of what is seen are carried to the mind, and it is here that understanding takes place. It is in the mind that the symbols are recognized, associations made, information processed and interpreted—based on the reader's knowledge and experience that he brings to whatever he is reading. These may or may not be similar to the author's. This is why different interpretations of books and poems occur among readers. Each reader has his own unique fund of knowledge and background of experience that influences his interpretation of whatever he is reading. The teacher who expects every student in a class to come up with the same answer to the routine question, "What is the author saying in that poem?" should perhaps substitute the question "What is *your* interpretation of this poem?"

How Does One Read?

Contrary to what many people assume, our eyes do not flow smoothly across the page as we are reading. Instead, our eyes move in a series of jumps and pauses.[6] These are called saccades and fixations. We only read during the fixations—not when the eyes are moving. When the eyes pause, they take in a portion of visual information (about six or seven items) which is fed into our short-term memory, sometimes called our working memory. This is a sort of holding station where the visual information is processed by the brain. Our working memory is of limited duration. We must give attention continually to this information or we lose it and while this is going on we cannot attend to anything else. It is as though there is a "shut-down" in our vision while the brain is processing this information.

What happens to this portion of information taken in? If the brain can organize the information and wants to keep it, then the information is transferred into our long-term memory for permanent storage, but recall is not always instantaneous. Sometimes this can be frustrating to us, say, when we want to remember the name of our child's second grade teacher or the author of a particularly interesting book or the name of a special restaurant.

The dyslexic has serious problems with both short-term memory and long-term memory. Words must be recognized and information organized for the information to be transferred to long-term memory. If what he is trying to read makes no sense, he tries again, and usually his short-term memory becomes overloaded because there is a limit to the amount of visual information that the brain can handle at any one time. Since the maximum is six or seven items, if the dyslexic is trying to "sound out" the individual letters of a word and this results in nonsense, then he has to try again. If unstable letter and word forms change in appearance and if he takes too much time in trying to figure out the word, his short-term memory bogs down. The brain cannot process the nonsensical information fed to it. Furthermore, stress and fear of making a mistake can get in the way of thinking and cause visual-memory overload.

This often happens when the dyslexic student is asked to read aloud in front of the whole class.

What the dyslexic already knows and has experienced (sometimes called nonvisual information[7]) plays a part in short-term memory and helps him make sense of what he sees and thus stores in his long-term memory. The effort itself, this trying so desperately to make sense of reading, contributes further to a very slow reading rate. Figure 2.1 illustrates the relationships of the components of the memory system discussed here.

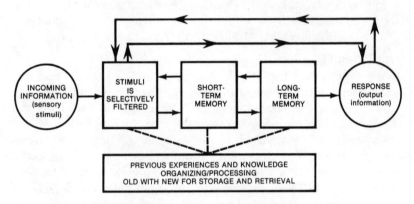

Figure 2.1.The relationships of the components of the memory system.

It is common for dyslexics (as well as other retarded readers) to have many regressive eye movements—when the eye goes back to get another look, to try again. Frequent regressions contribute to poor comprehension, lack of fluency, and slow reading.

His problem with short-term memory affects the ability of a dyslexic to copy accurately from the chalkboard, the overhead projector, charts, or books. It affects his ability to keep a visual image or auditory image of a reading or spelling pattern long enough for it to become internalized and transferred into long-term memory. And, remember, it affects any task involving listening as well.

The major problem with long-term memory is in retrieving specific information quickly at a certain time. In many cases, the dyslexic student may not provide an answer to a particular question, written or oral, as quickly as the teacher wishes, and she may turn to another student for the answer, thinking that the dyslexic student does not know it.

Both short-term memory and long-term memory problems can also affect the dyslexic's performance on timed achievement tests.

Understanding Writing

Writing is another form of communication by language. The author is attempting to convey his thoughts to the reader by means of words. Writing is related to both spoken language and reading, but it is not the same. In our country, from ocean to ocean, throughout various geographical regions, citizens speak with various dialects. An educated or uneducated Southerner will speak somewhat differently from an educated or uneducated Midwesterner or New Englander. Residents of New York speak differently from their close neighbors in New Jersey (listen for those dropped "r's" in New York). And, in fact, within each state there exists a variety of dialects.

In the United States, no one regional dialect is recognized as being *the* national standard. Each geographical region has its own regional standard, but while citizens across our country may speak quite differently, this does not prevent us from reading and understanding the same national newspapers, or magazines, or books on the best-seller lists. We even watch and understand the same national television programs.

What does writing do? It cuts across all the many different dialects, for the conventional form of writing can be read by those who might find another's speech a little difficult to understand. *Writing is a kind of language melting pot for all the variant types of speech.* It is an important form of communication and a significant part of our education; therefore, it should be a major part of the curriculum in our schools.

What is Involved in Writing?

Contrary to what some think, writing is *not* the mirror image of reading. Like reading, writing is actually a complex process, but it is a different ball game from reading. The writer must recall the correct spelling of a word and then encode the word, forming it from the individual letters that make it up. The writer has to recall the exact form of each letter and the sequence in which these letters occur. Does the word begin with a capital letter? Is it a hyphenated word? Must it be underlined? The *t*'s and *x*'s have to be crossed and the *i*'s and *j*'s dotted. Then there must be a space between the individual words and the appropriate punctuation must be chosen—a period, comma, question mark, and so on. Not only do the letters have to be in correct sequence to form a word, but the sequence of the words in a sentence must be considered.

What skills are needed for writing? One must have a good visual image (revisualization) of the spelling of the word, as well as of the formation of the letters that make up the word, and the capacity to recall these from memory. There are no "silent" letters in spelling! All letters in a word must be written. A sense of sequence is needed for the letters and words to appear in the right order. It is also needed for the orderly development of ideas and the organization of thought in whatever is being written. And the writer must have understanding of the purposes of punctuation so that the reader will be able to

17

make sense of the material. Recall—retrieving information out of one's long-term memory so as to have something to write about and relating it to other types of information and experiences—must be done in any writing.

The dyslexic's problems with unstable letter and word formations, his confusions with visual and auditory sequencing, and punctuation, and his difficulty in retrieving information from his long-term memory storage in a short time—all contribute to his poor writing abilities.

What about phonics for spelling? Isn't it essential in order to spell correctly? Some may think it heresy when I say that students who "spell by ear" are the poorest spellers. Yet, it is true. The following is a letter that shows the types of spelling errors often made by students who have overly depended on phonics and who have been taught to spell by "ear."

> Deer Miz Jonsun,
>
> Thay tel me u ar a good teecher. I wont too hav u for my teecher nex yeer. Becauz I hav truble with reeding and riting and speling. Sum uv my teechers tryed too teech me wurds and I had a grate deel of fonix evri day. Wun teecher sed she wuz going too beet fonix n my hed and she wurked hard and I ges she did a thoro job and now I hav truble understanding whut I reed and peepul laf when thay see how I spel wurds. Pleez teech me nex yeer and help me too reed and spel rite.
>
> I luv u,
> Bob

To spell correctly, the spelling of words must be *remembered*. Stressing the relationships of the meaning of words will help here and will help children to internalize what they know about their language and how words are related. Gradually, developmentally, they will apply this knowledge to their spelling of words and acquire a stock of correctly spelled words. This is how the dyslexic must build up a vocabulary of words to use in his writing. The association of meaning with the word will help him much more than any phonics sounding of letters that at times may vary (to him) in shape as well as sound.

The matter of spelling is treated more fully in Chapter Seven, where it is pointed out that children's spelling progresses through a series of stages and that certain types of spelling errors are normal for young children.[8] As they mature, so too does the development and accuracy of their spelling and writing.

People are often surprised when they hear that the pronunciation of words is a very unreliable guide to spelling. How often do we hear teachers or parents telling children to "sound it out" when students ask for help with spelling a word! Yet one-third of the words in a standard dictionary have more than one accepted pronunciation. A majority of the words in our language have "silent" letters (as the *k* and *w* in *know* or the *e* in *bake* or the *a* in *beat* or the second *e* in *beet*). One-sixth of the words contain double letters (as in *kitten, bottle,* or *correct*). Many different spellings can be given for most sounds. For example, the vowel *e* has at least ten vowel sounds. The long sound of the vowel *e* can be spelled fourteen ways, only one-fifth of the time with the *e* alone.[9,10] No wonder dyslexics, especially auditory dyslexics, have so much trouble with vowel sounds! Teaching the vowel sounds admittedly "is undoubtedly the most difficult and confusing part of an entire phonics program."[11] Difficult and confusing for *any* child, not just a dyslexic child! Clearly, phonics cannot insure correct spelling.

Take the word *work*: If a teacher asked a student to "use your phonics" to spell *work*, the child might write *wurk, werk, wirk, wurc, werc, wirc, wurck, werck, wirck*—none of which correctly spells the word *work*, but all of which are pronounced the same as *work*.

To illustrate the peculiarity of English spelling, George Bernard Shaw constructed the word, *ghoti*. This word is pronounced *fish*. Why? The *gh* combination is pronounced like the *gh* sound in *cough* (which is an *f* sound), the vowel *o* is pronounced like the *o* sound in *women* (which is the short *i* sound), and the *ti* combination is pronounced like the *ti* in the word *nation* (which is a *sh* sound). Hence: *ghoti* is pronounced *fish*.[12]

Let's be sensible about teaching spelling. Let's not further disable our dyslexic child by turning him into a "phonics misspelling cripple."

Understanding Speaking

The human vocal apparatus can produce an almost infinite variety of speech sounds for sending words from a speaker to the listener. These have different acoustic patterns caused by the various kinds of articulatory movements used to produce them. Articulation is the process by which the shape of the vocal tract is changed to produce the various sounds.

But speaking is more than just producing speech sounds, more than mere talking. Speaking requires thinking and involves imagination and a sensitivity to the listener. Good speech is produced with ease and confidence and is pleasing to the ear. The tempo as well as the volume is suited to the listener.

An individual speaks because he has something to say to someone. He has some information he wishes to share. Or an opinion he wants to give. He may have a question to ask. Or an answer to a question asked. Whatever the case, he has something to say, and so he speaks.

In school, it is not the student who does most of the speaking, but the teacher. Actually, teachers need to do less talking and more listening. How else can the students' speaking skills improve? Students need to be encouraged to talk freely with one another in class discussions, in planning a joint project or activity. The object of conversation is to share ideas, and students should have opportunities to present these ideas in logical order, to respond to the ideas of others, and to make suggestions.

Dyslexic students are often quite willing to talk, and, if their self-esteem has not been shattered, will work in groups and make contributions to class discussions. What they have to say is usually based more on their background of knowledge and experiences than on their textbooks, unless they have been given material which they can read with understanding. Sometimes the fund of information which dyslexics have acquired is remarkable in view of their reading problems, since reading is one way to acquire new knowledge.

If, however, you pay close attention to what is being said, you will note that the ideas and events expressed by the visual dyslexic are usually out of sequential order. In school, their verbosity sometimes helps them to get around requirements and slip through the grades. The auditory dyslexic, on the other hand, is not as glib and does not have as great a range of speaking vocabulary as the visual dyslexic. And he may not enunciate clearly; his speech frequently may include spoonerisms, twisted syllables, and the like. Both visual and auditory dyslexics often find it hard to recall the right word when needed because of difficulties in retrieving information quickly from long-term memory.

Understanding Listening

Hearing is not the same as listening. We hear with our ears but we listen with our minds. Listening is more complex than hearing and involves a knowledge of the language, relating what is heard to past knowledge, and making sense out of it. Listening requires giving active and conscious attention to the speaker. It requires thinking, reacting, and associating ideas.

Students in school spend at least 45 percent of their time listening to instruction. Imagine! This much time just listening in the classroom—not participating really in what is going on—just listening. But listening is an active process. Hearing may be inactive, but listening requires involvement on the part of the listener. The good listener *thinks* as he listens and is not distracted from listening. He controls his emotions as he listens to what is said, and he recognizes his responsibility in affording courtesy to the speaker. Because he is thinking as he listens, he is able to react, to respond to what he has heard, or to think of additional information to add to a subject. Good listening is an active, not a passive skill. The listener must pay attention to the words, phrases, and ideas presented by the speaker.

If the material presented by the teacher is interesting or useful to the students, if it means something to them, then they will attend to what is being said. If it is not, they will not. It is as simple as that.

Teachers sometimes, unwittingly, contribute to nonlistening habits when they pitch their instruction at a level higher than the listening level (understanding) of their students, or when they have students who have difficulty reading material aloud, stagger through a textbook or story, repeating words and hesitating, so that what they are reading drags on the mind of the listener.

On the other hand, parents and teachers, no matter the difficulties, must listen attentively to youngsters when they have something to say to them and must serve as listening models for the children.

The visual dyslexic may be a somewhat better listener than the auditory dyslexic who finds the sounds of language confusing and inhibiting; but the sequencing of thoughts and the retention of ideas is faulty in both. Indeed, because dyslexics tend to be sensitive to the sounds of their environment, many have had to learn to shut them out, to develop a kind of insulation against the distractions of noise. This sensitivity to noise and movement combined with the difficulties of processing language make dyslexics faulty listeners.

The Language Arts

Reading, writing, speaking, and listening are all interrelated. The words of our language are a common bond between them. While reading and listening are the "receptive" components of the language arts, and speaking and writing are the "expressive" components, all require an active participation on the part of the student.

In our everyday life, we tend to speak more than we listen or read, and we read more than we write. On the average, people retain only 50 percent of what they hear (no matter how hard they concentrate), and two months later they generally remember only 25 percent of what they have heard.[13] Elementary school students retain even less. One wonders whether the "lecture method" of instruction in our schools is ever as effective as some believe.

The dyslexic student nearly always has trouble in any lecture type situation. His faulty information-processing system responds better to demonstrations, student-participation exercises and activities than to lectures or textbook reading—in all subjects.

Notes for Chapter 2

1. Walter T. Petty and Julie M. Jensen, *Developing Children's Language* (Boston: Allyn and Bacon, 1980), p. 21.

2. A. L. Rowse, "Why a Contemporary Shakespeare?" *King Lear* (Lanham, Maryland: University Press of America, 1984), p. 6.

3. *Picturesque Word Origins* (Springfield, Mass.: G. & G. Merriam, 1933); H. L. Mencken, *The American Language* (New York: Alfred A. Knapp, 1980); A. L. Rowse, *Introduction in the Contemporary Shakespeare Series* (Lanham, Maryland: University Press of America, 1984—.)

4. Dominic V. Massaro, "Language and Information Processing," *Understanding Language,* Dominic V. Massaro, ed. (New York: Academic Press, 1975), p. 5.

5. Richard L. Venezky, "Regularity in Reading and Spelling," *Basic Studies on Reading,* Harry Levin and Joanna P. Williams, eds. (New York: Basic Books, 1970), p. 42.

6. Edmund Burke Huey, *The Psychology and Pedagogy of Reading* (Cambridge, Mass.: The MIT Press, 1908/1968), pp. 15–50.

7. Frank Smith, *Reading Without Nonsense* (New York: Teachers College, Columbia University, 1979), p. 33.

8. There have been a variety of studies concerning the developmental nature of students' spelling progress. You may wish to read further in: J. Richard Gentry, "An Analysis of Developmental Spelling," *GNYS At WRK, The Reading Teacher* 36 (November, 1982), pp. 192–199; "Learning to Spell Developmentally," *The Reading Teacher* 34 (January, 1981), pp. 378–381; Edmund H. Henderson and James W. Beers, eds., *Developmental Learning to Spell, and Cognitive Aspects of Learning, A Reflection of Word Knowledge* (Newark, Delaware: International Reading Association, 1980).

9. Bradley M. Loomer, *Educator's Guide to Spelling Research and Practice* (Des Moines, Iowa: Iowa State Department of Education; Iowa City, University of Iowa, 1978), p. 18.

10. Ernest A. Horn, "Spelling," *Encyclopedia of Educational Research,* 3rd ed. (New York: Macmillan, 1960), pp. 1338, 1342–1343.

11. Arthur W. Heilman, *Phonics in Proper Perspective,* 5th ed. (Columbus, Ohio: Charles E. Merrill, 1985), p. 65.

12. Lincoln Barnett, "The English Language," *Language Arts in the Elementary School,* Hal D. Funk and DeWayne Triplett, eds. (Philadelphia: Lippincott, 1972), p. 103.

13. Stanford E. Taylor, "Listening," *What Research Says To The Teacher* No. 29 (Washington, D.C.: National Education Association, 1964), p. 4.

PART TWO: THE LANGUAGE DISCONNECTION, DYSLEXIA

The dyslexic, whether visual or auditory, can look at the word and hear the word. The language disconnection occurs as the brain sees and listens and attempts to make sense of the symbol or sound.

—A. M. H.

CHAPTER

3

OVERVIEW OF THE COMMON CHARACTERISTICS OF DYSLEXIC STUDENTS

Whatever you cannot understand, you
cannot possess.
—*Goethe*

To be able to call a demon by its name
is halfway to getting rid of him.
—*André Maurois*

This and the following two chapters on the characteristics of dyslexia are offered to help parents, classroom teachers, and principals develop some understanding of the nature of dyslexia and of the numerous problems dyslexics have in coping in the classroom, in the home, and in the world in which they must live from day to day. With deeper understanding and knowledge should come a realization that these children are in special need of supporting, caring adults who are willing "to go the extra mile" to help them overcome their difficulties and to give them the encouragement and acceptance for which they yearn.

This is *not* intended to qualify nor enable anyone to diagnose dyslexia. (That will be the subject of a separate book.) Parents should not attempt to diagnose dyslexia. Neither should regular classroom teachers nor other school personnel who have not had the appropriate training.

Parents and teachers should, of course, be alert to the characteristics and symptoms of dyslexia, and if dyslexia is suspected (and the child is at least eight years old), steps should be taken to have the child tested for the disability. Use your common sense when observing a child suspected of being dyslexic. Ask yourself if his behavior is really atypical, not that of the "normal" child. Keep a record of your observations and the child's behavior. Keep samples of the child's work: writing, drawings, math, social studies, science, spelling, exercises in reading, and written records of general classroom and playground behavior. Does he need to have directions repeated? Does he make errors when copying from charts or the chalkboard? Has he recently had his vision and hearing checked? Keep all this information in a special folder with his name on it and give it to the person who will be examining the child.

Calling a Spade a Spade

When a student has been diagnosed as being dyslexic—and we do not arrive at this diagnosis without compelling evidence—this must be so stated in order for the child to receive the appropriate treatment. I often think of Mark Twain's answer to the oft-repeated question: "Who *really* wrote Shakespeare's works?" His flippant reply was "They must have been written by some other fellow named Shakespeare." So, too, with diagnosing dyslexia. Mark Twain might in this respect have said to the skeptics, "There's no such thing as dyslexia. That ailment is some other condition called dyslexia." And Shakespeare would probably join in with, "What's in a name? That which we call a rose by any other name would smell as sweet."

As for me, I say with Meander (343–292 B.C.), "I call a fig a fig, a spade a spade." When a child has dyslexia, let's say so. If he doesn't, let's not.

The Three Categories of Dyslexia

During the past fifteen years, I have found that the dyslexics with whom I work tend to fall into three categories, or groups, of dyslexia[1]: visual, auditory, and a combination of visual and auditory dyslexia. Visual dyslexia is by far the most common type. Sixty-one percent of my cases have been visual dyslexics, 20 percent have been auditory dyslexics, and 19 percent have been a mixture of both. When a student has a combination of both visual and auditory dyslexia, the visual component is usually, though not always, more pronounced than the auditory.

Characteristics Common to All Three
Categories of Dyslexia

There are certain characteristic problems that occur with all types of dyslexics. At the same time, there are certain reactions to these problems by the dyslexic, his parents, and his teachers that typically occur, usually as a result of not knowing that the student *is* dyslexic, or not understanding the nature of the condition. The following pages should help pinpoint specific difficulties and illustrate how the dyslexic, his parents, and his teachers have responded in such situations. I hope the result will bring about a modification of attitudes and expectations, and a deeper empathy for what is happening to the dyslexic child.

Slow Work Rate

The dyslexic child usually works very slowly. He is the student who fails to finish his seatwork and often is kept in during recess with firm instructions from his teacher "to finish that work!" Yet day after day this recurs. What the teacher must understand is that the student cannot help this slow rate of work. He is not necessarily a lazy child. He does not need to be "pushed." And he should not be punished by having to stay in the classroom while his classmates go outside to run and jump and play and exercise their muscles and socialize. He needs the break even more than the other children because of the pressure to perform—which he feels constantly.

Often the dyslexic child must take home the work he does not finish in school with instructions to get it done by the next day. This means the child cannot play outside after school—ride his bicycle, run around, climb trees—and exercise, which he needs to grow and to develop normally. Here again, he is being denied opportunities to grow physically, socially, and emotionally, to learn the give-and-take of neighborhood friendship. In a way, this is a form of punishment for parents, too, as one or the other usually has to sit with the child and give him the help that he needs in order for him to complete the work.

So what happens? The dyslexic child feels resentment at what he considers unfair treatment. The parents feel resentment that they must put aside necessary chores, or ignore the crying baby or the other children's questions, or miss a favorite television program, in order to help the dyslexic child with his seatwork. Once in a while, perhaps—but *every* day? The parents resent their child for not "doing what he is supposed to be doing in school." And they resent the teacher for not teaching him so that he does not have to do his work at home. The teacher in turn resents the child for "not doing his work" in spite of all the usually successful tactics she has used. And of course she resents the parents for "spoiling" him. All these feelings of resentment add pressure and tension to an already bad situation. I wonder. Could this fall under the category of "cruel and unusual punishment"?

What to do? First of all, the world will not collapse if teachers reduce the quantity of work. Let the student work ten math examples instead of twenty-five. Let him write half a page instead of two or three, answer five questions instead of ten. Make sure that any work that he is expected to do on his own is on his independent (free reading) level; that is, that he miss no more than one or two words out of about one hundred words in a narrative passage. And be sure that he understands what he has to do. Work an example out with the child to ensure that he understands what is expected of him. Praise him when he does the work well. And always keep in mind, it is the teacher's job—not the parents'—to "teach" new words, new skills, and other concepts included in the school curriculum.

Even if the work is at the appropriate level for the dyslexic student, even if he has been previously prepared for it, he will still work more slowly than his classmates—not because he is less intelligent than the others but because it takes more time for him to integrate and process the information; that is, to make sense out of what he is seeing and writing.

Timed School Tests

The dyslexic student knows that he works slowly. He cannot get through his work quickly enough nor produce the necessary quantity of work to please the adults in his life. He tries hard, but his best is never good enough. He never seems to be able to catch up with what has to be done. He is constantly feeling the pressure of time and of work. One dyslexic phrased it quite aptly: "I feel as though I am on a treadmill, going around and around and around without ever having a chance to stop and catch my breath."

When the student with dyslexia is faced with a standardized achievement test that has time limits, and the teacher is standing in front of the room with a stopwatch in her hand, he is likely to panic. Anxiety inhibits his thinking. It increases as the teacher announces, "You have fifteen minutes left . . . Now you have only ten minutes to finish. Work fast! Five minutes left! Four . . . Three . . . Two . . . ONE! All pencils down!" At that the dyslexic is ready to jump out of his seat and explode.

Following Oral Directions

Following oral directions can be difficult for the dyslexic, and so he asks his teachers and parents to repeat what they have said. This constant need for repetition can get on the nerves of both teachers and parents if they are not aware of the reason that prevents the student from following directions the first time around. It is common for the dyslexic to be told, "If you would just pay attention and listen the first time you would know what to do!" But "just paying attention" is not the major problem.

The visual dyslexic has difficulty remembering a series of directions because of both his sequencing problems and his short-term memory problems. The auditory dyslexic has trouble because of his particular difficulties in processing and understanding what has been said to him. This affects sequential auditory organization. Both types of dyslexics end up with bits and pieces of directions that become jumbled and confused in their minds. And so the directions are not followed as given.

The following directions by a classroom teacher were recorded at the time given:

> It's time now to put away your seatwork and get out your math books. Turn to page 81 and look at the word problems on that page. (Turning to a student:) No, Mary, you can't go to the bathroom now. Put your hand down and pay attention. On page 81 . . . (Pointing to another student:) Johnny! Get back in your seat and get out your math book. Now, I want everyone to work the first five problems at your desks, then some of you can come up to the board and show the rest of us how you did your problem.

Directions such as these would confuse any student, but imagine how utterly lost the dyslexic child can become. He knows that he must ask the teacher to restate the directions, and she will probably be cross as a result. Sometimes dyslexics develop the survival technique of pretending to turn to the right page in the book and then peeking at a friend's book to find the correct page. If he gets caught, he may be warned to "keep your eyes on your own work!"—or worse. He may even be accused of trying to cheat—which can have a devastating effect on a child who is valiantly trying to do what he is supposed to be doing.

What about his home life? Here the dyslexic has the same trouble when his parents tell him to finish his supper, and after that to be sure to feed the dog, to empty the trash basket, to hang up his jacket which he left on the living room sofa, and to pass the biscuits, please. When these chores are not done—or only one or two are done—and he neglects to pass the biscuits, he is scolded for not listening or for being lazy.

Neither the teacher nor the parents intend to be unkind to the dyslexic child. Such behavior on their part is usually due to their not knowing that the child is dyslexic, and thus not understanding his inability to behave normally.

Lecture Instruction and Note-Taking

Lecture instruction is the least effective method of teaching for any student. For the dyslexic, the results are dismal. Both visual and auditory dyslexics have trouble with lectures for the same reasons they have difficulty in following directions. Both have processing problems, either because of difficulty in following sequence and development of ideas presented, or because of auditory confusion over what was heard. As a result, note-taking is unsatisfactory—

full of incomplete sentences, scraps of ideas, events out of order. The notes provide little or no help in studying for tests and examinations.

Unless the dyslexic condition of the student is discovered and helped before he reaches middle school or high school, where teachers more often use the lecture method, he can become overwhelmed by life at school and his failure to achieve. Unless he gets help from someone quickly, he is likely to withdraw from school—psychologically or physically.

Sensitivity to Sound and Movement in the Environment

As mentioned above, dyslexic students tend to be sensitive to what is going on around them and are easily distracted. Noise and movement can divert their attention. This characteristic, of course, varies with the individual student, but clearly the "open classroom" concept *as applied in America* with the on-going noise and movement in the large rooms without walls is not for the dyslexic student. Neither is a "departmentalized" type of schooling where students move from class to class, period to period, throughout the day. The young dyslexic always feels the pressure of time hanging over him, the need to get his work done before the bell rings; and then he hurries off to the next class only to have the same thing happen all over again. It is unfortunate that so many of our elementary schools have jumped on the departmentalization bandwagon in an ill-advised mimicry of the high schools. It would be far better for the dyslexic student if he did not have to face departmentalization before high school.

The *traditional self-contained classroom* where children are with one teacher all day is the best arrangement for the student with dyslexia. In such a classroom, the teacher gets to know the students so well—their strengths and weaknesses, what makes them "tick,"—that she is able to plan instruction in flexible blocks of time on a more individualized basis. I am referring to the regular classroom of this type, not the special education classroom for handicapped students. I make the distinction because I suggest that the dyslexic child *can* function in such a situation if the teacher understands the nature of dyslexia and is willing to make certain adaptations in her expectations and instructions. Here, in a regular self-contained classroom, the dyslexic student feels more secure and less pressured. He does not continually have to adjust to different teacher personalities and other students as he changes classes during the school day while fighting that tyrant, the clock. He is more able to concentrate on applying himself to learning.

Sounds in Isolation Phonics Instruction

Both visual and auditory dyslexics suffer when they are taught the phonic elements *in isolation rather than in a meaningful framework of words and context*. You will recall that in the last chapter *meaning* was considered the critical element in working with the dyslexic student. Dyslexics already have severe problems in organizing and integrating information and making sense of what they try to read. They do not need any more roadblocks thrown up by nonsensical teaching. Words broken down into individual letters "sounded" in isolation are much more difficult to learn than when they appear as a meaningful entity. Why? A letter sounded in isolation has no meaning and sounds like gibberish. The crucial element of meaning is not there.

I do not say that phonics should not be taught; I do say that it should not be taught in a way so as to compound the dyslexic's problems. Most of the basal reader series (books designed especially for the teaching of reading), while emphasizing phonics instruction, do *not* instruct teachers that *r* says *er* or *ruh* or *rur*, or that *l* says *el* or *luh* (as teachers have been heard to tell their students). What nonsense! When a teacher tells a child that *b* says *buh*, *a* says *ah*, and *t* says *tuh*, the child comes up with *buhahtuh*—which is absurd. Sometimes, teachers will tell students to "say it fast" thinking that this will help with the blending of the sounds. What actually happens is that the child says *buh-ah-tuh*, *buh-ah-tuh*, *buhahtuh* resulting in a three-syllable nonsense word for the one-syllable word *bat*. (No wonder such children have trouble with syllabication!) The child might end up with the words *batter* or *butter* or *barter* for the word *bat*, which will make hash out of what he is reading. Such instruction for the dyslexic child can be disastrous.

As Doris J. Johnson of the Department of Communication Disorders at Northwestern University and Helmer J. Myklebust, well-known scholar in language, psychology, and neurology, and also at Northwestern University, have pointed out, when a vowel sound is added to the consonant (or blend or digraph), as illustrated above, "it is nearly impossible for children to blend sounds into words."[2] They relate this experience with a child: "An eight year old tried to sound out the word *pat* and said, 'puh-a-tuh—puh-a-tuh?' What does that mean?"[3] Nothing. Meaningless. And a typical reaction to this kind of instruction. Yet how often does one hear from teachers (and parents, probably quoting the teacher) that "Johnny knows all his sounds. His problem is, he just can't *blend* them." Or, this statement: "Johnny knows all his sounds. His problem is not with phonics. It's his *comprehension*. He just doesn't seem to understand what he reads."

The dyslexic child has enough trouble with comprehension without adding the sounds-in-isolation barrier. Such instruction also results in slow, labored reading—another problem the dyslexic already has—and excessive lip movements.

How do children learn? They tend to "chunk" meaningful units. By chunking, I mean grouping items. For example, it is far easier for a child to "chunk" meaningful words than isolated letters. And since they can "chunk" up to six or seven items at a time, more words can be read in this manner. Is it not better to take in six or seven words than six or seven individual letters that may or may not make up one word?

Any program that advocates teaching the sounds of letters in isolation should be avoided at all costs for the dyslexic student, whether his affliction is visual or auditory. A child *can* learn to read in this way, but (1) his progress will be ever so much slower, (2) his comprehension will be poor, (3) his reading will be slow, (4) his fluency in reading will be poor, and (5) he will likely develop the habit of lip movements.

The Notes for this chapter provide some comments by eminent educators concerning the teaching of sounds in isolation.[4]

The critical ingredient in any instruction of the dyslexic child must be to emphasize meaning. Dyslexic students are already handicapped in school. Let's not be guilty of making phonics cripples of them, too.

Reluctance to Read Aloud

After so many problems in reading, so many mistakes made when reading aloud in front of the class, the dyslexic has naturally developed a fear of performing in front of his classmates and his teacher. He knows that he will make mistakes, say the wrong words, and read in a halting and repetitious manner. He knows that when he reads aloud, his classmates do not enjoy listening because of his faltering manner and use of incorrect words, which make it hard for them to follow the thread of thought. These fears come to the fore and create feelings of anxiety so that he even misses words that he *does* know. Panic takes over. If you observe closely you can notice his flushed face, rapid breathing, clenched hands, stilted posture.

Unfortunately for the dyslexic, there are still some teachers who use the "Round-Robin" technique to teach reading—each student takes a turn reading aloud from a book—although this is not the recommended procedure suggested in the basal reader teacher's manual. Nor is this taught to prospective young teachers by up-to-date professors in the teacher-training colleges, because of the problems it can cause even normal students. It is the least effective way to teach reading. It also demands the least preparation, the least imagination, and the least effort on the part of the teacher.

Some upper elementary, middle, and high school teachers use the Round-Robin technique when "teaching" science or social studies or other subjects. Down one row and up the next, the students take turns reading aloud from their textbook. (This is "teaching?") The excuse often given for this procedure at the upper levels of school is that, "The textbook is too hard for some of the students and this is how to make those students know what's in the book." Sometimes, the teachers ask for "volunteers," and so the same capable students end up reading in class day after day. (And what is this telling the other students?)

But we know the problems the dyslexic already has with listening and retaining information. When the pressure and anxiety of being called on to read the textbook aloud, in front of others, is added, no wonder the dyslexic tries to find some way out—leaving the room or creating a diversion or just plain refusing and thus invoking the wrath of the teacher.

Reluctance to Write

The dyslexic student has had trouble with his spelling and his handwriting since the beginning of his school years. So many papers have been returned to him covered with red ink and corrections that he has developed a way to cope with the increasing demands of writing—he writes as little as he can, and when he does he uses the words he thinks he can spell. For example, when asked to write about his favorite animal he may want to write *dinosaur* or *elephant* or *squirrel*, but instead he will write *cat* because he knows he can spell that word. (He may avoid *dog* because of the unstable *d* and *g*, but if he does he is likely to capitalize the *d*.) His most enjoyable movie may have been *Amadeus*, but when asked to write about this topic, he may write *Star Wars* instead because of the simpler spelling. Results of some tests and inventories, where the dyslexic student must fill in blanks to answer questions or finish incomplete sentences, are invalid for this reason. The substance of what he has written appears immature, of course, and his sentences are usually choppy or of the run-on kind.

The following story was written by a student in our summer clinic:

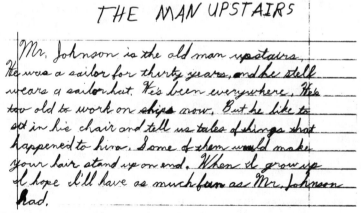

Fig. 3.1   Example of Keith's writing

How old do you think Keith was when he wrote this story? In what grade would you place him? Would you say his intelligence is at a low level, average, or above average level?

Keith's story is included here as an example of how a low stock of spelling words can affect a student's writing. His writing appears fairly neat, with only ten strike-overs and two misspelled words (*stell* for *still* and *like* for *likes*). At its highest, the readability level of this paragraph would be beginning third grade. Most of the words used are one-syllable words; it is the length of the sentences that makes the readability level as high as it is. Is this the writing of an eight-year-old child in the third grade?

Hardly. It is the writing of a high school auditory dyslexic who had learned to circumvent those red corrections on papers by using words that he was fairly certain he could spell correctly—but which in no way indicated the capability of Keith. When he wrote this story, Keith was almost eighteen years old and in the eleventh grade—with an IQ of one hundred twenty-five.

The dyslexic has learned that another way to cope with the demands of writing is to copy from books rather than give the information in his own words. He may make some mistakes in his copying, but the errors will be far fewer than if he had written on his own. He finds a survival technique in plagiarism that helps to make his life run more smoothly. It is another way to help him get from day to day.

In a way, these self-protective "coping" devices have made the dyslexic student act dishonestly in setting down what he truly thinks and truly feels. Yet he is basically as honest as any other child, and so, this, in turn, increases his feelings of guilt and lowers his self-esteem.

Hyperactivity

Is hyperactivity a common characteristic of dyslexia, as often claimed in articles and books on the disability? Are all dyslexics overactive, full of energy, constantly in motion, excessively talkative, into everything?

The answer is no. This may be symptomatic of certain brain damage and can even be symptomatic of an emotional disturbance, or of certain physical diseases. Such characteristics may be the result of frustration, boredom in class, or even a particular learning style. Dyslexics, however, are not necessarily hyperactive; some are and some are not.

In a study of five hundred dyslexic children, ages six to eighteen, only 26.8 percent were found to be hyperactive, 22 percent of them boys and 4.8 percent girls. (And 13.8 percent of the boys and 4.6 percent of the girls were found to be *hypoactive*; that is, lethargic, lacking energy.[5])

One Category: A Combination of Visual and Auditory Dyslexia

Some children have a combination of visual and auditory dyslexia. My experience has been that usually the visual dyslexia is more pronounced than the auditory dyslexia, though the reverse may be the case at times.

I have found 19 percent of the dyslexic cases diagnosed at the clinic to be a combination of both types. It would seem that having one kind of dyslexia is enough of a burden without being saddled with both kinds, but it does occur. In such a case, depending upon the severity, the prognosis is less encouraging. But, these children *too can be helped.* It is harder to alleviate the difficulties and it takes longer. The residual remnants of difficulties tends to be stronger, and it is to be expected that some difficulties may be lasting to a certain degree.

"Sam" came to the College Reading Clinic when he was eight years old (with a mental age two years higher). He had repeated the first grade and was now scheduled to repeat the third grade. His instructional reading level—that used by the teacher for the formal teaching of reading with his basal reader—was first grade. His independent or "free reading" level was preprimer, which is the first step above readiness. His dyslexia had not been diagnosed prior to his coming to the clinic. He had a combination of both kinds.

The following is a copy of Sam's story which he wrote after the Fourth of July holiday:

It took Sam twelve minutes to write the story. When he had finished, he was asked to read what he had written. This is what he wrote:

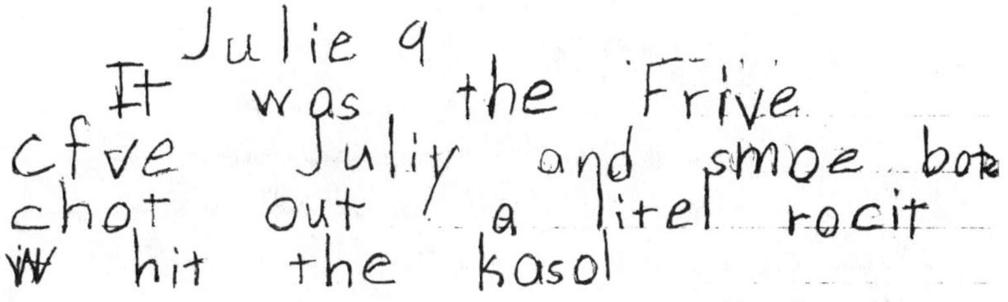

Fig. 3.2   Story written by Sam, C.A. 8-6, M.A. 10-6.

This is what he read:
> It was the fourth of July and somebody shot out a little rocket. It hit the castle.

When "Jack" came to us for help with his reading and writing problems he was nine years old, with the mental age of a fifteen year old. His instructional reading level was at the primer level. Like Sam, his dyslexia had not been diagnosed prior to his coming to the reading clinic. He, too, had a combination of visual and auditory dyslexia.

Jack was asked to write about something that he especially enjoyed, and he wrote the following story about his Honda. After he finished writing it, his teacher asked him to read what he had written and she taped what he said. Later, she wrote what he had said below his story (See Figure 3.3).

Children such as Sam and Jack definitely require remediation on a one-to-one basis, as frequently as can be arranged (and afforded) in order to make the most progress. Progress will be slow, but with hard work on the part of the

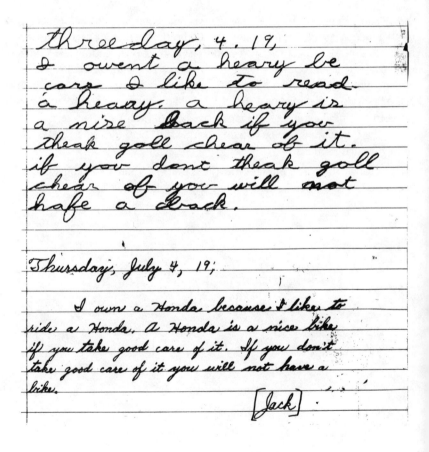

Fig. 3.3   Story written by Jack, C.A. 9-1, M.A. 15.0.

specialist and the student, with the cooperation of the parents and teachers, such students *can* accomplish a great deal.

The following two chapters will deal specifically with the particular characteristics of visual dyslexia and auditory dyslexia as different categories of dyslexia.

A Word About Dysgraphia

Dysgraphia is sometimes spoken of as being another type of dyslexia. It is a disorder of visual-motor integration—the hands and eyes working together smoothly. The handwriting of a child with dysgraphia can be difficult to read and at its worst is said to resemble "chicken tracks."

Yet the "symptoms" of dysgraphic handwriting apply also to the handwriting of the visual and auditory dyslexic. Their writing may be hard to read because of their problems with visual memory in copying, in spelling, in writing, in retrieving visual images or trying to match auditory images of sounds with the printed letters. The dyslexic's handwriting is slow and laborious. His writing is usually filled with corrections, strike-overs, and erasures. Their papers are usually messy in appearance.

Other than being a result of visual and auditory dyslexia, poor handwriting can also be the result of finger agnosia, which is a kind of short-circuit in the neural pathways from the brain to the fingers (or vice versa). A child with finger agnosia produces poor letter formation, insecure writing with letters of varying size and spacing, strike-overs, and frequent erasures. The writing rate is slow, and writing is a laborious task. A child with finger agnosia might show no other symptoms except poor handwriting and certain types of misspellings and reversals in words.

Students thought to have dysgraphia have been referred to me (with no mention of dyslexia or finger agnosia). Yet the symptoms of dysgraphia were caused by the dyslexia or finger agnosia—or both, for a dyslexic can also have finger agnosia.

I question the existence of dysgraphia as a separate entity and suggest that it is either a manifestation of an existing dyslexic condition or of finger agnosia. Of course, certain types of injury to the writing hand could affect a child's handwriting, but this would be because of the injury rather than dysgraphia.

Notes for Chapter 3

1. Notes on categories of dyslexia:
    (a) Ingram, in his discussion on the nature of dyslexia, speaks of three kinds of dyslexia: some predominantly "visuospatial" in type, some predominantly "audiophonic," and others a combination. Thomas T. S. Ingram, "The Nature of Dyslexia," *Early Experience and Visual Information Processing in Perceptual and Reading Disorders* (Washington, D.C.: National Academy of Sciences, 1970), pp. 412, 431, 437.

(b) Ingram, Mason, and Blackburn in a retrospective study suggest three categories: visuospatial, audiophonic, and one with "correlating" difficulties. From their description, it would appear that the third category corresponds with my third type of a combination of visual and auditory dyslexia. Thomas T. S. Ingram, A. W. Mason, J. Blackburn, "A Retrospective Study of Children With Reading Disability," *Developmental Medicine and Child Neurology* 12 (1970), p. 273.

(c) Johnson and Myklebust describe two major types of dyslexia: visual and auditory. They do not mention a combination of visual and auditory as a third type, although they state that " . . . dyslexia is rarely found in isolation. Other disabilities are manifested as a part of the total syndrome." They also describe the writing disorder called dysgraphia and the math disorder called dyscalcula. Doris J. Johnson and Helmer R. Myklebust, *Learning Disabilities, Educational Principles and Practices* (New York: Grune and Stratton, 1967), pp. 150, 152–271.

(d) Later, in 1978, Myklebust speaks of visual dyslexia, auditory dyslexia, and an inner-language dyslexia. He refers to inner-language dyslexia as *word-calling* and says usually there are deficiencies in both auditory and visual verbal processing (combination type). He says that the letters and words are perceived and the child can say them (because he can "read"), but the level of meaning is bypassed. Helmer R. Myklebust, "Toward a Science of Dyslexiology," *Progress in Learning Disabilities* IV, Helmer R. Myklebust, ed. (New York: Grune and Stratton, 1978), pp. 15–16.

(e) Jordan describes the three kinds of dyslexia as being visual, auditory and dysgraphia. No mention is made of a separate combination subtype, although note was made that "few children are handicapped by only one form of dyslexia." Dale R. Jordan, *Dyslexia in the Classroom,* 2nd ed. (Columbus, Ohio: Charles E. Merrill, 1977), pp. 1–9.

(f) Aaron and Bakes have found three groups in their work with college students who have "specific reading disabilities." These are called the Acoustic Short Term Memory Deficient Group, the Visual Short Term Memory Group, and the Lexical Access Deficient Group. P. S. Aaron, and Catherine Bakes, "Empirical and Heuristic Bases for Diagnosis and Remediation of Specific Reading Disabilities," *Topics in Learning and Learning Disabilities: Issues in Reading Diagnosis,* 2, (Gaithersburg, PA: Aspen, 1983), p. 37.

(g) Boder also reports on three subtypes: visual, auditory, and mixed. Those with visual channel problems she calls *dyseidetic* (Gestalt-blind), those with auditory channel problems she calls *dysphonetic,* and the mixed group is called *dysphonetic-dyseidetic* (or *alexia*). In contrast to my findings, more of her dyslexics fell in the auditory group, with less in the visual group. However, her study has been criticized for questionable diagnostic assessment procedures involving a word recognition task and its determination of gestalt or phonetic approach through timed versus untimed responses, the spelling test of known and unknown *reading* vocabulary words for visual and auditory classification, and the possibility of interpreting such errors in other ways. For example, *rough* is an irregular word. Why would a child be expected to sound this out? The word *doubt* has a silent *b*. Visual recall is what is needed with these irregular words. Other interpretations of behaviors can also be questioned. Samples of errors analyzed were small. Any of these could affect the placement of a dyslexic into a particular group. And no diagnosis of dyslexia should be made on the basis of a spelling test alone. Many excellent readers are poor spellers and her selection procedures could include nondyslexic as well as dyslexic children. A word of caution: there have been several studies using Boder's system. The validity of such studies and conclusions should be weighed carefully. Elena Boder, "Developmental Dyslexia: A Diagnostic Approach Based on Three Atypical Reading Patterns," *Developmental Medicine and Child Neurology* 15 (1973), pp. 663–687. Elena Boder, "Developmental Dyslexia: A Diagnostic Screening Procedure Based on Three Characteristic Patterns of Reading and Spelling," *Learning Disorders* Vol. 4, B. Bateman, ed. (Seattle, Washington: Special Child Publications, 1971), pp. 297–342. Elena Boder, "Developmental Dyslexia: Prevailing Diagnostic Concepts and a New Diagnostic Approach," *Progress in Learning Disabilities* Vol. 2, Helmer Myklebust, ed. (New York: Grune and Stratton, 1971), pp. 293–321. Elena Boder, "Developmental Dyslexia: A New Diagnostic Approach Based on the Identification of Three Subtypes," *Journal of School Health* 40 (1970), pp. 289–290.

2. Johnson and Myklebust, op.cit., pp. 157–158.

3. Ibid., p. 158.

4. Notes on Phonics Instruction, Sounds in isolation

    (a) "In approaching each phonic element, deal only with words as units, not sounds isolated from words. If possible, employ words already in the reading vocabulary of pupils as examples of the letter-sound association in teaching each element." George D. Spache, *Diagnosing and Correcting Reading Disabilities*, 2nd ed. (Boston: Allyn and Bacon, 1981), p. 250.

    (b) "Originally, the sounds of individual letters were taught but mainly in the last decade linguists have pointed out that letter-sounds are never produced singly but in the context of words, and that usually the positioning of the letter determines its particular sound. If individual letters are sounded there is a tendency for *uh* to be added, so that one gets the distorted pronunciation *huh*, *ruh*, and *guh*. When the sounds of individual letters are 'blended' or synthesized, one gets the words *bat* sounding more like *barter*, which can be very confusing to some children." Elizabeth J. Goodacre, "Methods of Teaching Reading," *The Reading Curriculum* Amelia Melnik and John Merritt, eds. (Morristown, N.J.: General Learning Press, 1972), p. 118.

    (c) "While materials account for many of the errors found in phonics instruction, teachers sometimes contribute errors quite on their own. Certainly, this is so of teachers who have been heard saying to children that the sound of *r* is *er*; that the sound of *l* is *ul*; that the sound of *fr* is *fur*; and so on." Delores Durkin, "Phonics: Instruction That Needs to be Improved." *The Reading Teacher* 28 (November 1974), pp. 152–156.

    (d) "It is true that one cannot separately pronounce letter sounds, which taken together constitute the pronunciation of English words, and children are not asked to do so. They are taught that a particular letter represents the same speech sound in many different words, and they are invited to think or sub-vocalize this sound when the letter occurs in a word they are attempting to solve." Arthur W. Heilman, *Phonics in Proper Perspective*, 5th ed. (Columbus, Ohio: Charles E. Merrill, 1985), p. 10.

(e) "Word-attack skills must be taught as a first-aid to meaning. Words must be introduced in a communication context so that, as the reader moves along, meaning clues to recognition may also be a first-order, functional source of help. Phonics must be taught in a pronunciation unit or in context, but not in isolation." Russell Stauffer, "Dictated Experienced Stories," *The Reading Curriculum* Amelia Melnik and John Merritt, eds., op.cit., p. 155. (Also University of London Press)

(f) " . . . in my judgment children who believe they can read unfamiliar words just by 'blending' or 'sounding' them out are likely to develop into disabled readers, the type of secondary students who are condemned for being 'functionally illiterate' because they do exactly what they have been taught and try to read by putting together the sounds of letters. Besides, I think it would be difficult to exaggerate the complexity and unreliability of phonics. To take just one very simple example, how are the letters *ho* pronounced? Not in a trick situation, as in the middle of a word like *shop*, but when *ho* are the first two letters of a word? Here are eleven common words in each of which the initial *ho* has a different pronunciation: *hot, hope, hook, hoot, house, hoist, horse, horizon, honey, hour, honest*. Can anyone really believe that a child could learn to identify any of these words by sounding out the letters?

"Incidentally, the preceding illustration underlines an important requirement of phonics that is never explicitly taught at school—that phonics requires reading from right-to-left. The eleven different pronunciations of *ho* that I have just given all depend on the letters that come next." Frank Smith, *Reading Without Nonsense* (New York: Teachers College, 1979), p. 56.

5. Edith Klasen, *The Syndrome of Specific Dyslexia* (Baltimore: University Park Press, 1972), pp. 67, 71, 193–194.

CHAPTER

4

VISUAL DYSLEXIA

True wisdom consists not only in seeing
what is before your eyes, but in foreseeing
what is to come.
—Terence

In the little world in which children
have their existence, whosoever brings them
up, there is nothing so finely perceived and
so finely felt, as injustice.
—Charles Dickens

A child is not a visual dyslexic because of any loss of vision. We *look* with our eyes, but *it is our brain that sees and makes sense of that which is seen*. A visual dyslexic has difficulty with processing and interpreting the images received by looking. Light rays from whatever it is we are looking at pass through the cornea of our eye, and on through the pupil, the lens, the vitreous humor (the soft, jelly-like material that maintains the shape of our eyeball), until they reach the retina which is the inner layer of the eyeball occupying about four-fifths of the inner circumference of the eye and situated toward the rear of the eyeball. The following illustration of the eye will help in understanding the location of the various parts.

PARTS OF THE EYE

The human eye is a complex organ. The part we normally see, *left*, is only about one sixth of the complete eye, *below*.

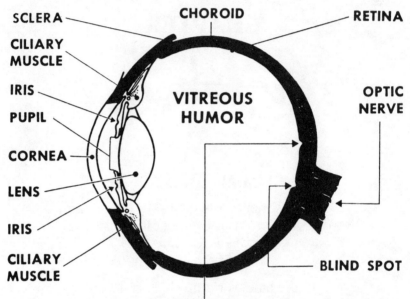

FOVEA CENTRALIS—AREA OF SHARPEST VISION

Fig. 4.1 The parts of the eye. (From "Eye," by John McWilliams, *World Book Encyclopedia,* Vol. 6, Chicago: Field Enterprises Educational Corporation, © 1968, p. 359. Used with permission.)

When light strikes the sensitive cells of the retina, it stimulates nerve cells. Messages then flow along the optic nerve to the *visual cortex,* which is the "seeing" part of our brain.[1,2] The brain must now do something with these images; it must make sense of them by classifying, organizing, relating and making associations, and integrating them with knowledge that has been stored previously in the brain. This is a process of interpretation, and it is with this process that the visual dyslexic has trouble.

Parents and teachers need to know that several types of vision defects can create symptoms similar to those of dyslexia. For example, *nearsightedness* (myopia) results in blurred distant vision. A student with this defect can have trouble copying correctly from the chalkboard, or the overhead projector—as does the visual dyslexic. Students who are *farsighted* (hyperopia) will find close seatwork and reading in books fatiguing and will likely try to get out of these tasks whenever possible—as does the visual dyslexic.

With *astigmatism*, vision tends to be blurred and distorted. Such a vision problem will cause a child to tire easily and avoid close work or prolonged copying. Letters and words that are similar in form are often confused. Reversals may occur. The student with astigmatism will experience difficulty in any sustained reading task. Headaches are common. Most of this behavior is also typical of the visual dyslexic.

Muscular imbalance (strabismus) can cause a blurring of letters and words, and even double vision in severe cases. The same word (or letter) may appear differently at different times. Lines of print may be jumped over. A word in one line may be transferred to a line above or below (insertion errors). Again, these too are symptoms of visual dyslexia.

Lack of fusion and *aniseikonia* (the lens of the two eyes are not in focus) can cause readers to mix letters in words (transpositions), to make reversals, to lose their place, and to read very slowly. Sounds like dyslexia, doesn't it?

One can understand that certain eye defects can affect the accurate assessment of a child's problems and can affect a student's performance not only in his reading class but in other subjects as well. Any student who is having trouble with reading and writing should have a complete vision examination by an eye doctor.

This is not a chapter on diagnosis. I shall not attempt to discuss in detail other problems that can cause symptoms similar to those of the visual dyslexic. This is simply a plea for common sense, for not jumping to conclusions when certain types of errors occur in reading and writing. For example, I have heard very often parents and teachers make an automatic and often unwarranted assumption in such statements as, "Johnny reversed his letters (or words) and he must have dyslexia." Pause and consider the following possible reasons for reversal problems, other than dyslexia:

1. Could the child possibly have an eye defect?
2. Has he had sufficient left-to-right orientation? We read and write in a left-to-right direction, but this does not come naturally to children. Primary teachers should spend a good amount of time in this area.
3. Is the child a left-hander? Left-handed children need much more training in left-to-right orientation than right-handed children. It is common for young left-handers to reverse letters and to begin writing from the right side of the page (mirror writing).
4. Are the words or letters reversed quite similar in appearance? The child may need more visual discrimination work. The words *was* and *saw* or *no* and *on* have the same shape. Perhaps the child needs to learn to direct his attention to the

distinguishing features of such words and letters—to consider what makes them different from one another.

5. How old is the child? Visual immaturity can cause reversal errors of letters and words, as well as visual discrimination types of mistakes. (This is discussed more fully in Chapter Seven concerning early identification of dyslexia.)

6. Is it likely that self-consciousness, anxiety, worry, stress, or fatigue are causing the child to make reading and writing errors similar to the dyslexic patterns?

7. Is the child expected to read in a book that is too difficult for him?

Sequencing Difficulties

The inability to understand the sequence of things and events is a major problem of the visual dyslexic. He has difficulty with the sequencing of letters in words, with learning a series, such as the order of the letters in the alphabet from *A* to *Z*, the days of the week, the months and seasons of the year, sets of numbers in series, the progression of time on the clock, and the score by innings on a baseball scoreboard.

The months of the year (Figure 4.2) were written by Roger, a visual dyslexic, age nine years and ten months. Roger was to repeat the fourth grade in the fall.

Roger was asked to write the months of the year "in order, beginning with the first month of the year." As you can see he began with October and wrote November and December, skipped to March, skipped to June, July, August, then jumped back to January, then to August (spelled another way this time), and September. He omitted February, April, and May.

The visual dyslexic may at first appear to be fluent in retelling a story, but listen carefully and you will note that he has trouble relating the events of a story in the order in which they occurred, or predicting outcomes, or making inferences about what has been read. The main idea of a story may escape him altogether.

Indeed, the visual dyslexic usually has difficulty relating the incidents in his own life in correct order. For example, he may tell you that his dog died last month (when it was a year ago), and that he went to the circus a year ago (when it was only a month ago). He has problems with chronology in history and with the order of steps in a science laboratory experiment or the logical steps in proof of a theorem in geometry.

This flaw in sequencing is why the visual dyslexic has trouble following oral directions. It is also the reason he has trouble following any written directions of several steps. Baking a cake or making a souffle requires a sequence of actions that can frustrate the visual dyslexic. If given a kit for con-

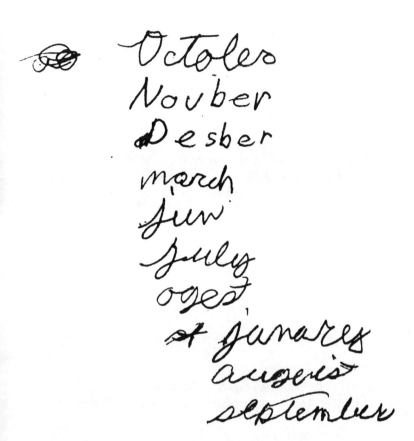

Fig. 4.2   Months of the year written by Roger, a visual dyslexic.

structing model airplanes or toy automobiles, he will probably begin assembling the pieces right away rather than first reading the written directions. The adult dyslexic, when faced with assembling his new lawn mower or a new bicycle for his child, will proceed immediately by trial and error—and common sense—with the unused directions often blowing away unheeded.

A young visual dyslexic may like to play catch with his dad in the backyard, enjoying the companionship and attention of his father, but games such as baseball can be confusing because of the sequence of plays and calls and the need to grasp visually what is going on in the game, let alone keeping track of the score by innings. Sports of this type usually have a low priority in the visual dyslexic's life, although he may "mouth statistics" with the guys, which helps him to be part of the group. He is likely to prefer sports such as fishing or hunting or swimming.

Working jigsaw picture puzzles can be frustrating. There is a sequence of development in joining the various pieces of a puzzle. Visual imagery is important in such a task, and visual dyslexics have difficulty relating the parts to the whole. Visual analysis and synthesis are hard for them.[3]

In school, taking multiple-choice tests and examinations can throw the visual dyslexic into a panic because of the requirements for sequence, recall, and visual memory.

Because of his poor visual memory, he has trouble copying from any of the materials used by teachers in instruction. For, when copying, the visual dyslexic makes mistakes in spelling, omits certain punctuation or capital letters, and may even skip a line of writing, even though the model is there in front of him. Teachers often find this hard to understand, and they display their impatience—"there it is, right in front of your eyes!"

Figure 4.3 is a story copied from a chart by Mark, a nine-year-old visual dyslexic. He took ten minutes to copy these lines, and still did not complete the entire story.

This is the original from which he was to copy:

Bob and Dan saw Sam Watts walking on the dock. The three men stopped.
"See the big ship?" asked Sam.
"Sure did!" Bob and Dan said. "Must be a mile long."
Bob and Dan saw Sam was in a hurry. "Got to run," Sam said. "See you!"
"Sure," said Bob and Dan. "See you, Sam."

Observe Mark's intermixing of cursive and manuscript writing as well as of capitals and lower case letters. Note the various errors:

In the first sentence, he
— reversed the final letter *b* of *Bob*, so that it appears to be a *d*,
— added an additional *n* in *and*,
— substituted a *d* for the *n* in *Dan*, so that the word appears as *Dad*,
— originally reversed the beginning *s* of *saw* but corrected it by writing over the reversed letter,
— omitted the word *Sam* altogether (or did he omit *saw* and write *Sam* as *saw*, reversing the *m*?),
— wrote *Watts* as *watts*, with the *w* in lower case,
— omitted the word *walking*,
— wrote *dock* as *Dock*, with the *d* capitalized,
— had no space for the period, so he placed it at the beginning of the next line.

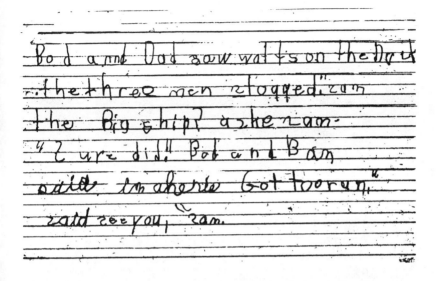

Fig. 4.3 Story copied by Mark, a visual dyslexic, from a chart.

In the second sentence, he
> — did not begin the sentence with a capital *T*, but used the lower case *t* instead,
> — reversed the *s* and the two *p*'s in *stopped*.

In the third sentence, he
> — continued on the same line as the second sentence instead of beginning another paragraph,
> — began and ended the sentence with *zam* for *Sam*, with the *s* reversed and not capitalized,
> — wrote *big* as *Big*, with the *b* capitalized,
> — omitted ending quotation marks,
> — reversed the *s* in *asked*,
> — omitted the final *d* in *asked*,
> — placed the period at the level of the top of the *m* which it followed.

In the fourth sentence, he
> — reversed the *S* in *Sure*,
> — ran his exclamation and quotation marks together,
> — wrote *Bob* as *Bod*, with the final *b* reversed,
> — wrote *Dan* as *Ban*, substituting *B* for *D*.

In the fifth sentence, he
> — omitted *Bob and Dan saw Sam was*,

— wrote *a hurry* as *aberie*, the two words joined as one, with the
er substituted for *ur* and *ie* substituted for *y*,
— omitted the period.

In the sixth sentence, he
— omitted beginning quotation marks,
— added an *o* to *to* (*too*),
— misplaced *Sam* at the end of the sentence, with the *s* reversed
and not capitalized,
— omitted the period,
— omitted beginning quotation marks,
— substituted a comma for the exclamation mark,
— wrote the closing quotation marks in the opposite direction.

Mark did not copy the last sentence.

Such errors are typical of a visual dyslexic's far point copying. He also
has trouble copying the questions from the end of a chapter of a book. The frequent instruction, "Copy the questions at the end of the chapter and then answer them for homework," becomes a laborious task for the visual dyslexic
student. He will also find difficulty in drawing what he sees at the end of a mi-
croscope in science class, or copying a map in social studies class.

Drawings of the Visual Dyslexic

The visual dyslexic has difficulty describing accurately his bedroom or
house or classroom, and when asked to draw them, items of furniture, windows, and doors often are omitted or misplaced and out of proportion. Indeed, his drawings as a whole tend to be poor and lacking in details. Whether
the picture is of a room, flower, tree, or human being, it appears to be the
work of an immature child.

Figure 4.4 shows a visual dyslexic's self-portrait. This child was nine
years old at the time. Note the omission of such details as the nose, mouth,
ears, eyebrows, hair, and items of clothing. Also note the lack of proportion of
the figure as a whole—head, hands, trunk, legs, and feet.

Figure 4.5 is an example of a self-portrait of an older boy, age fourteen.
More details are included in the face, but the ears are missing. And while he
has drawn his belt, other details of his clothes are missing so that the drawing
appears to be that of a belted nude on a skateboard! Note the insecurity of the
drawing—the erased lines, the strike-overs.

Figure 4.6 is a drawing of the room where a visual dyslexic and his
teacher work. The boy was ten years old. He had been working in this room
each weekday morning for four weeks. The teacher took him to another room
in the building and asked him to draw a picture of the room where they
worked. He was asked to try to make it look just like the room.

You can see that many details are missing. He did include the round table and the two chairs, marking his particular place. Another chair and a triangular table are included, but bookcases, other tables lining the walls and pieces of furniture are omitted. The window is drawn out from the wall and is greatly out of proportion. Another window is missing. An arrow indicates the

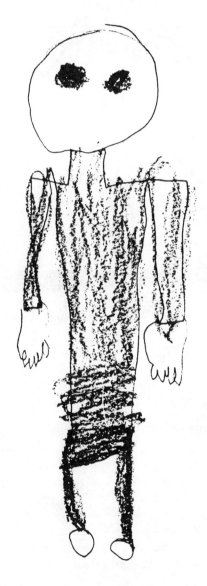

Fig. 4.4 Self-portrait drawn by a visual dyslexic, age nine.

door where he erased part of the line to make a door. Notice the insecurity of the lines, the strike-overs, the incorrect strokes.

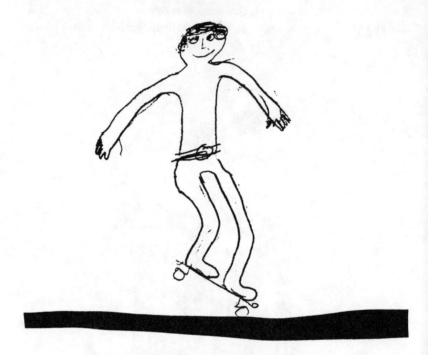

Fig. 4.5   Self-portrait drawn by a visual dyslexic, age fourteen.

The visual dyslexic, of course, has trouble with his visual memory—with revisualizing (picturing in his mind) how something or some place looks. Hence the lack of details, the incorrect proportions, the omission of objects, the insecure lines—all of which result in immature and unrealistic drawings.

Irregular (Unpredictable) Words

Irregular words, sometimes called unpredictable words, give the visual dyslexic student a great deal of trouble because these words must be *visually recalled* since they are exceptions to the phonics rules or have letters that are not pronounced (silent letters). Thus, phonics provides little or no help with these words. Examples of such words in our English language would be *once, one, does, ought, bough, cough, though, rough, break, are, night, gnaw, know, love, their, eyes, to, mother, father* (not *fat her*)—and hundreds more. The student must store a visual image of these words, both for

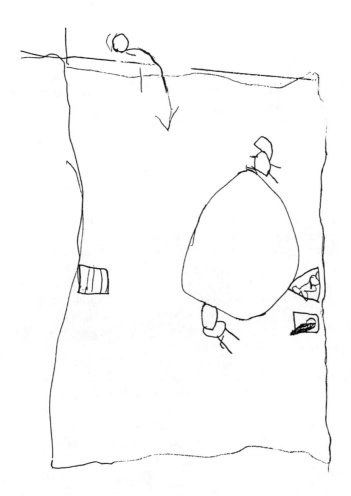

Fig. 4.6   Sketch of remedial classroom by a visual dyslexic, age ten.

reading and for spelling. Then he must revisualize, picture in his mind, how these words appear, and apply this to what he is reading or spelling.

Words with the diminished vowel stress (called the "schwa")—where any vowel can take the sound—as the *o* in *button* (but ʹən), the second *e* and the *a* in *elephant* (el'əfənt), or the *i* and second *e* in *president* (prez'ədənt) present huge barriers to a dyslexic in reading and spelling certain words correctly.

Visual Discrimination Errors/Reversals

Letters and words similar in form are likely to be confused or reversed at times. A child may confuse *b* with *d* or *was* with *saw*, but not all the time. Some authors of books and articles on dyslexia have erroneously referred to a dyslexic's problem as "reading backwards" or "writing backwards." This is not the case, or all the letters and words would be reversed, and reading could be learned simply by learning the reversed letters. What does occur is an inconstancy, an instability of form. It is common for the visual dyslexic to capitalize certain letters in writing so as to circumvent this inconstancy of form. You will recall that Mark wrote the word *big* as *Big* and *dock* as *Dock*. Dyslexics may write *baby* as *BaBy* or *bad* as *Bad*. Usually it is not the last letter that is capitalized.

Confusion with words such as *got/get, house/horse, want/went, tam/tan, how/now*, are typical of the visual dyslexic. Confusing words such as *bad/dad, big/dig, god/dog, pan/nap, saw/was* and *no/on* are also common for the visual dyslexic. Did you note the reversed letters and words in this second group?

I have found that the following letters give the visual dyslexic the most trouble. The letters within each set tend to be confused with one another:

b-d-p-q-h	t-f-j	M-W, m-w
r-h-u-n	h-p-y	N-Z, S-Z
v-w-l-u	e-o-c	a-e
	r-c-s	

Look closely at the above letters. Note the similar features. Turn *N* on its side and you have a *Z*. You can understand how inconstancy of form will create such confusions at times.

Letters are not alone in being confused by the visual dyslexic. Numbers, too, can give him trouble. You may find that the visual dyslexic will also confuse:

2-5	6-9	3-E	7-f

Spelling

Just as in reading, irregular words give problems in spelling. The speller not only must remember which letters make up the word, and what these letters look like, but also the sequencing of the letters in the word. He must revisualize exactly what a particular word looks like and its specific components. The visual dyslexic will make errors in spelling of the same letters (listed above) as those that confuse in Visual Discrimination.

Figure 4.7 was written by Bobby, age nine and a half, and of above average intelligence. Note the reversed numeral 5 occurs three times.

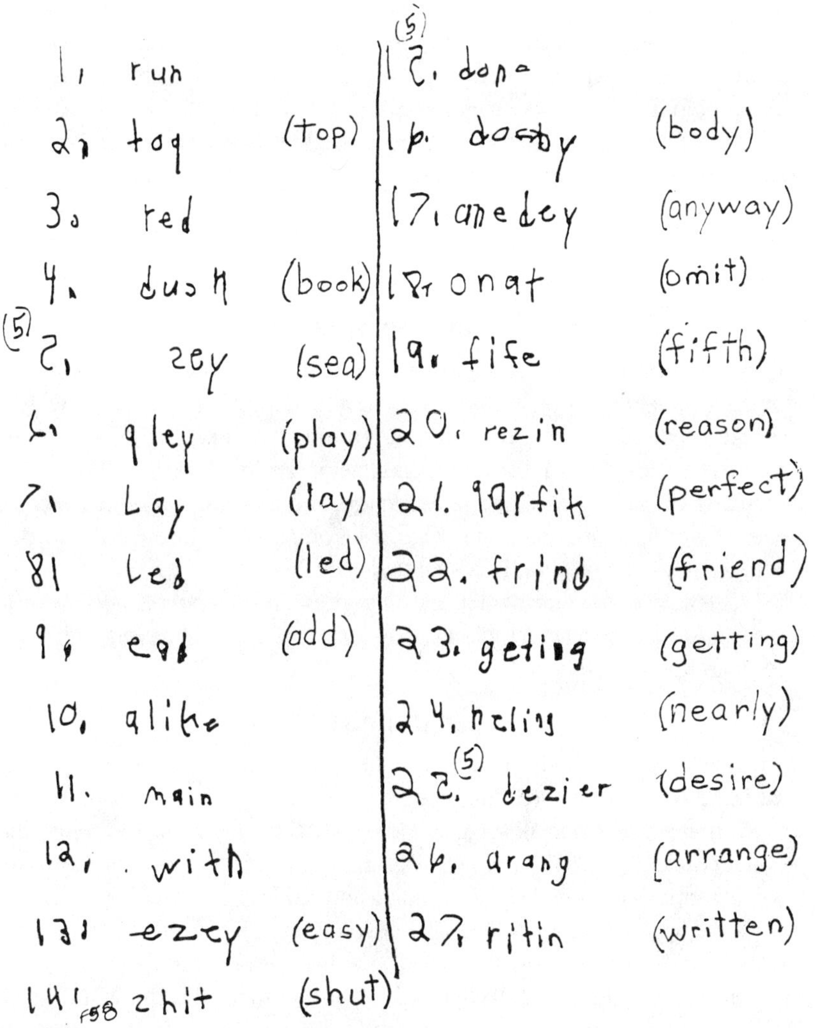

1. run
2. toq (top)
3. red
4. dush (book)
5. zey (sea)
6. qley (play)
7. Lay (lay)
8. Led (led)
9. eod (add)
10. alike
11. main
12. with
13. ezcy (easy)
14. zhit (shut)

(5)
15. dona
16. dooby (body)
17. anedcy (anyway)
18. onat (omit)
19. fife (fifth)
20. rezin (reason)
21. qarfik (perfect)
22. frind (friend)
23. geting (getting)
24. ncliy (nearly)
25.(5) dezier (desire)
26. arang (arrange)
27. ritin (written)

Figure 4.7   List of spelling words written by Bobby, a visual dyslexic, age nine and a half.

The visual dyslexic will write letters out of order in words (called trans-position errors). For example, he may write *left* for *felt*, *paly* for *play*, *who* for *how*, *pna* for *pan*, or *clam* for *calm*. Silent letters within words are often omit-ted and sometimes transposed. The visual dyslexic just cannot revisualize these words correctly in a consistent manner.

As I have already stated, these characteristics of the visual dyslexic are not being illustrated for diagnostic purposes, but only as a matter of informa-tion to help in better understanding his problems. I should note here, how-ever, that if a non-dyslexic child has been taught phonics by sounds in isola-tion, he may make certain errors typical of the dyslexic. Therefore, the method of instruction should be investigated before arriving at any final conclusions. (See Appendix A for examples of such errors, which have thrown some di-agnosticians off the track.)

Handwriting

Letter formation by the visual dyslexic is usually poor because of his in-constancy of letter forms, and his revisualization deficiencies. When he writes, his letters tend to be irregular in size, with frequent rotations, reversals, strike-overs as he tries to form the letters, and lots of erasures. There will be an in-termixing of capitals and lower case letters and of cursive and manuscript styles of writing. Mark's writing in Figure 4.3 on page 47 illustrates the incon-stancy of writing typical of the visual dyslexic.

It is easy to understand that learning shorthand symbols or coding sym-bols would be very difficult for a visual dyslexic to master. He has enough trou-bles with his own alphabet!

Arithmetic

The visual dyslexic will have trouble in arithmetic for the same reasons that he has trouble with reading, spelling, and handwriting. Language is nec-essary in math, as it is in all subjects. Here, words are often used to represent certain concepts. But number symbols and the operations on numbers are more specific than those used for reading and writing. The visual dyslexic has problems with arithmetical language development, just as in the "language arts."

Even if he could read all the words in the arithmetic directions and word problems, his sequencing difficulties would still affect his thought processes. He cannot organize the information given in the problem. Facts to do with simple addition and subtraction may be remembered, but the more complex tend to be forgotten. He may carry or borrow (regroup) the wrong digit. Mul-tiplication tables can drive him up the wall. Processes may be reversed while computing. Numerals may be reversed—a *2* may be changed to a *5* or a *6* to a *9*—which can result in major errors in calculation.

Referring to tables and bar graphs or copying geometric figures is likely to result in errors. His poor visual discrimination and unstable memory will cause the symbols for addition and multiplication (" + " and " × ") or the subtraction and equal signs (" – " and " = ") to be confused at times—just as with the letters *b* and *d* or *u* and *n*.

The vocabulary used in arithmetic, such as *quotient, subtrahend, associative*, and *product* are difficult for the visual dyslexic to understand and learn.

The concept of time is also hard to master. Learning to read time presents problems because of the sequencing of the numerals around the clock face and the visual dyslexic's reversal difficulties. He may read 6:00 as 9:00. Even if a child has a digital watch and he reads the numeral correctly, the digits may be transposed.

Social Studies, Science, and Other Subjects

Visual dyslexics have trouble reading maps and globes. The keys (legends) to maps are hard to use. They have difficulty reading any kind of floor plans. Estimating distance is difficult. They become confused with dates and times of events in history. They can get lost trying to create a time line as part of a history assignment. They even have trouble remembering the date of their own birthday, of other special family events, and of holidays commemorating famous people.

Some visual dyslexics may have an ear for music and be able to play an instrument, but reading the notes (or the words to the music) is another matter, depending upon the severity of the condition.

Standardized Reading Achievement Tests

Parents are often concerned about the scores of their child on the various standardized tests required by the schools. These require reading, of course, and any child with a reading problem is likely to score poorly although he may know the content asked. He may simply be unable to read all the words in the questions and so he cannot give the correct answer.

Teachers have wondered about the variance in reading achievement subtest scores. The visual dyslexic tends to score higher on the vocabulary subtest (usually consisting of finding synonyms or meanings for words) and lower on the comprehension subtest where he reads narrative passages and then answers certain questions. This is because of his sequencing difficulties and the confused order of the material in his mind. His memory weaknesses inhibit his looking back at the passage to try to find the answer. He has a hard time even keeping the question in his mind. He will probably give up and begin checking the answers in a random manner.

He is also likely to score higher on an oral reading test than on a silent reading test.

Oral Reinforcement When Working

The visual dyslexic will softly repeat words to himself as he works. He is drawing on his auditory modality to help him make sense of what he is reading. Even when he is asked to write the alphabet in sequence, he is likely to sing "The Alphabet Song" quietly to himself over and over—using it as a mnemonic device to help him recall the letters until he is finished. He may do the same when spelling words. (He is *not* trying to cheat or give away answers. He is trying to draw on a device to help him do what he has been asked to do.)

While it is customary for first grade children to use oral reinforcement (softly reading the words aloud to themselves) as they read, usually by second or third grade, children have moved into silent reading successfully, no longer using obvious lip movements (unless they have had Round-Robin instruction on a regular basis). This development is desirable, for one can read silently much faster than aloud. Comprehension tends to be better too.

But for the visual dyslexic we must make an exception. He needs to whisper the words softly to help him make sense of his reading and to serve as a self-correction help. This is his crutch. He needs it. Let him keep it.

Auditory Discrimination

The visual dyslexic usually has good auditory discrimination and can distinguish between similarities and differences in words when he hears them. His problem is with distinguishing between similar words when he *looks* at them.

Consonant Blends and Digraphs

When reading, the visual dyslexic is likely to transpose blends and digraphs, such as *three* for *there, gril* for *girl, calm* for *clam*, and *how* for *who*. But, as has been stated, one must be cautious here, for children who have been taught the phonic elements in isolation may have the same pattern of errors in both reading and spelling as dyslexics. (For example, if they have been taught that the blend *gr* says *gir* the child may read or write the word *grill* as *girl*.)

Configuration Word Recognition Strategy

Configuration refers to the shape of something. The shape of a word (or a letter) can be a clue to recognition, particularly if it is distinctive. Children tend to recognize the word *grandmother* rather easily because of its unusually long shape that begins with a letter dropping below the line. The word *ele-*

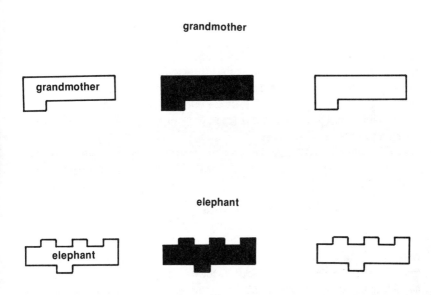

Figure 4.8   Shapes of words help in recognition of the words (configuration word recognition strategy).

phant is another word with a rather unusual shape and one which children learn easily. Figure 4.8 illustrates the concept of configuration.

The configuration word recognition strategy is of the visual type. The reader must "picture" the shape of the word in his mind—and do so very quickly to be effective. The visual dyslexic tends to have trouble making use of this clue to identify words because of his problems with revisualization.

Miscellaneous Problems of Orientation

In addition to problems with letter and word reversals, the visual dyslexic has a disorientation of time and space. He may draw heavily on his common sense, but still, this may not be enough in many situations.

The visual dyslexic child may be the one who remains on the playground after the others have returned to class. This is the child who "gets lost" in hide-and-seek games or "peeks" before the time is up. This is the student who, when sent with a message to the office, gets lost on the way. This is the child at home who does not "know when to come in for dinner." Or the child who, when his mother sends him to the neighborhood store with a list, arrives home two hours later without any satisfactory explanation. Where schedules are concerned, he seems to dawdle. If he attends a school where he must change rooms from class to class, he is often late (and may offer no reason, too embarrassed to admit he lost his way).

Teachers and parents find it hard to accept any of the visual dyslexic's explanations as to why he is late. What they must constantly remember is that the visual dyslexic *cannot help it*. He is not being deliberately disobedient. He is not a truant. He may seem not to care—but he does, very much. He knows these things are happening; he does not understand why; he would much rather that they not happen.

The same problems create difficulties in traveling—reading maps and getting around town, or across the country. The visual dyslexic can get lost—anywhere, any time.

Summary

The visual dyslexic's major problems are with sequencing, revisualization compounded by instability of letter and word forms, and other orientation difficulties. These can affect every school subject, many sports, his family relations, and the various community activities in which he may participate. They can affect any traveling he may do, which includes finding his way around his hometown and community.

Notes for Chapter 4

1. Stanley W. Jacob, Clarice Ashworth Francone, and Walter J. Lossow, *Structure and Function in Man* (Philadelphia: W. B. Saunders, 1978), pp. 312–314.
2. John R. McWilliams, "Eye," *The World Book Encyclopedia* (Chicago: Field Enterprises Educational Corporation, 1968), pp. 358–359; Morton F. Goldberg, "Eye," *The World Book Encyclopedia* (Chicago: World Book, Inc., 1985), pp. 358–367.
3. Doris J. Johnson and Helmer R. Myklebust, *Learning Disabilities, Educational Principles and Practices* (New York: Grune and Stratton, 1967), pp. 153, 156.

CHAPTER
5

AUDITORY DYSLEXIA

To children the whole isn't a collection
of parts, it's a complete unit. So,
paradoxical as it may sound, to go from the
whole to the part is to proceed from the
simple to the complex.
—*Kenneth Goodman*

When you know a thing, to hold that you
know it; and when you do not know a thing, to
allow that you do not know it: this
is knowledge.
—*Confucius*

A child is not an auditory dyslexic because of any loss of hearing. The auditory dyslexic often has keen hearing. We *hear* with our ears, but *it is our brain that listens and makes sense of what is heard*. An auditory dyslexic has trouble processing and interpreting the oral information which he hears.

How do we hear? There are three main parts of the human ear—the outer ear, the middle ear, and the inner ear. We actually hear sound deep inside the inner ear. Figure 5.1 illustrates the three major parts of the ear.

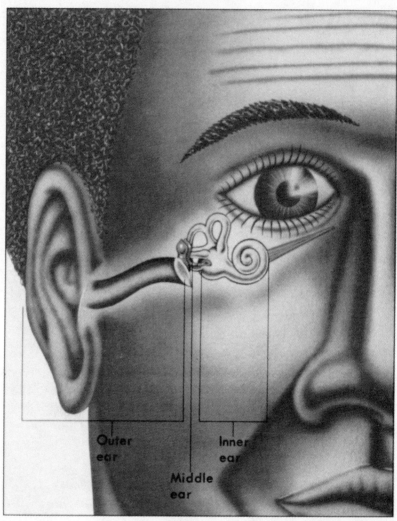

WORLD BOOK illustration by Colin Bidgood

The Human Ear extends deep into the skull. Its main parts are (1) the outer ear, (2) the middle ear, and (3) the inner ear.

Figure 5.1   The three major parts of the ear. (From "Ear," by David D. Caldarelli and Ruth S. Campanella, *The World Book Encyclopedia*, Vol. 6, Chicago: World Book, Inc., © 1985, p. 5. Used with permission.)

Sound waves (vibrations) can travel directly through the bones of our skull. The bones send the sound waves on to our inner ear. The outer part of our ear also collects sound waves in the fleshy curved, cuplike part attached to the side of our head (the auricle). These vibrations are directed into the hole or passageway (external auditory canal) and are guided to the middle ear through the eardrum—and a second eardrum if the first was ruptured at one time—on across three bones into the inner ear which has numerous intricate chambers and passageways. As the sound waves move along they cause the fibers (24,000 of them) which lie within the cochlea to move, and these fibers cause a vibration in specialized sense cells that make up the organ of Corti. The vibration of these sense cells (called hair cells) stimulates nerves that are attached to them. Messages flow through an auditory nerve to the center of hearing in the brain (temporal lobe) where the sounds are classified, processed, and interpreted.[1,2] Figure 5.2 illustrates how sounds travel to the inner ear.

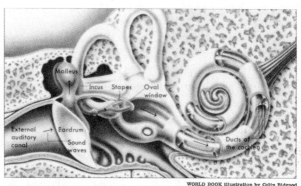

How Sounds Travel to the Inner Ear

Sound waves enter the ear through the external auditory canal. They strike the eardrum, causing it to vibrate. The vibrations flow across the malleus, incus, and stapes. The footplate of the stapes vibrates within the oval window, creating waves in the fluid that fills the ducts of the cochlea.

WORLD BOOK Illustration by Colin Bidgood

Figure 5.2   How sounds travel to the inner ear. (From "Ear," by David D. Caldarelli and Ruth S. Campanella, *The World Book Encyclopedia*, Vol. 6, Chicago: World Book, Inc., © 1985, p. 8. Used with permission.)

Parents and teachers need to be aware that abnormalities of the ear (or ears) can cause symptoms that are similar to some of those of an auditory dyslexic. Any child who is having academic problems in school should have his hearing tested with an audiometer by a trained examiner to determine if hearing defects may account for his difficulties.

Some school systems have a policy of regular screening for hearing problems. The person administering the test should be well-trained and skilled. Usually there is a speech and hearing clinic within driving distance where experienced examiners are available. Most cities have medical doctors who specialize in eyes, ears, nose, and throat who could give such hearing examinations.

What is so difficult about the ear is that a child can have normal hearing one week, then have an infection or injury, and suffer a hearing loss. Thus, parents and teachers need to be alert continually to the danger.

Disease or injury may cause partial or total deafness. Sound vibrations may be blocked by wax or foreign bodies that can lodge in either the external or the middle ear, or by adhesions of the bones in the middle ear. A ringing in the ear (Tinnitus) can affect hearing and may be caused by wax in the ear, holes in the eardrum, fluid in the middle ear (including water from swimming), and sometimes by taking drugs. Aspirin and streptomycin are two common drugs that could cause ringing in the ears.

Perforation of the eardrum can cause hearing loss, the extent depending upon the size and location of the hole. But even with almost complete loss of the eardrum, a person can hear slightly because of the sound waves that pass through the bones of the skull, bypassing the eardrum, to the inner ear.[3]

Children who have allergies, with stuffy noses and blocked eustachian tubes, can have temporary hearing loss of varying degrees.

Hearing loss can affect the auditory discrimination of students; that is, the ability to distinguish the minute differences in letters and words—as is the case with the auditory dyslexic. A child may not hear directions or instructions clearly, may not listen attentively because he hears only portions of what is said, and thus his interest wanders. Obviously, abnormalities in hearing can affect the correct diagnosis of a child and assessment of his performance in school.

If you have a child who is having problems with phonics, with structural analysis, taking notes, following oral directions, and paying attention to what is being said, consider the following before you refer him for possible auditory dyslexia:

1. Has he had a recent head injury or ear infection?
2. Could he possibly have a hearing loss?
3. Does he have frequent head colds?
4. Does he appear to have allergies?
5. Have you considered the possibility of a wax build-up in his ears?
6. Has he frequently been absent from school, and thus missed specific instruction in auditory activities such as phonics and syllabication?
7. Is the seatwork assigned him for these auditory activities at a level which he can read easily? That is, when new skills are taught, is there follow-up material that will not itself provide a block to the application of the new elements taught?

8. Is the child taking any kind of drug such as aspirin or streptomycin or any other?

In the chapter on visual dyslexia I spoke of the difficulty of *revisualizing*, or remembering and "picturing" words and objects and places formerly seen. The auditory dyslexic has difficulty in *reauditorizing*, remembering and "hearing" the sounds and sound patterns formerly heard and then applying them to his reading and spelling. When he looks at a word, he may be unable to say it even though he knows what the word means. For this reason, he will read silently better than orally. He can associate the word with meaning but cannot change the visual symbol of the word to the auditory.[4]

Let us hope that the auditory dyslexic does not have a classroom teacher who uses the Round-Robin technique to teach reading or other subjects, nor that his teacher assigns oral reading for homework—stories to be read aloud each evening at home. He needs to read silently at these times. Oral reading should be limited to diagnostic and remedial purposes.

Auditory Integration and the Dyslexic

The auditory dyslexic has trouble with certain intrasensory auditory functions, such as distinguishing between the sound units of language and synthesizing them into words, or taking a word and dividing it into parts like syllables. As a result, he cannot learn if taught by a synthetic (sounds in isolation) approach to teaching the phonic elements. He has trouble perceiving the relationship of the sounds of language with those represented by print; that is, matching the sound of the word with the printed word—or matching the phoneme (sound of a letter) with the grapheme (the letter as we write it).

Phonics and spelling rules are almost meaningless to him. So too are the diacritical markings used in dictionaries to designate the pronunciation of words.

Auditory Discrimination

The many disorders in auditory discrimination make it very difficult for the auditory dyslexic to make sense out of what he is hearing and trying to read. One of the major limitations caused by auditory dyslexia is the inability to "hear" even minimally the similarities and differences in words and letters. For example, he may confuse the sound of *m* with that of *n* (as in *man* and *Nan*), the sound of *v* with that of *f* or *th* (as in vine, fine, and thine). The letters *b, d, t, p,* and *g* may sound alike to him. He may say that the words: *back, pack,* and *tack* are the same. He may not perceive that the words *boy* and *big* begin with the same sound, or that *got* and *not* end with the same sound.

The Vowels and Vowel Digraphs

Variations of the vowel sounds really throw the auditory dyslexic into a quandary. He is bewildered when trying to discriminate between the short and long vowel sounds, such as those heard in *fat* and *fate* or *bet* and *beat*. He confuses some short vowel sounds with others, such as those heard in *got* and *get*, or *pin* and *pan* and *pen*. He especially has trouble with vowel sounds when heard in isolated form, but when words containing certain vowel sounds are given in a sentence he can draw on context clues to help him make sense of what he is reading and predict the correct word.

The schwa vowel sound like the *o* in *button*, which any vowel may represent in certain words, is nearly impossible for him to distinguish. (Actually, teachers should not even attempt to teach this perplexing concept to the auditory dyslexic.) To make matters worse and even more confusing for this student, the vowels in our language copy other vowel sounds, such as the short *u* sound in *mother* (written with an *o*, not a *u*), or the short *o* sound in *watch* (written with an *a* not an *o*), or the *ai* in *said* which has the short *e* sound (but is not spelled that way).

The auditory dyslexic may spell the word *meet* in either of several ways—*met* or *meat* or *mete*. And then, too, he may spell *meat* as *meet, met*, or *mete*. His spelling can be truly appalling.

Phonics must be kept in proper perspective for the dyslexic student. Trying to "pound" phonic elements into his head will not make him proficient at spelling or reading. On the contrary, it will only add to the confusing bits and pieces of sounds already floating around in his head.

The Consonant Blends and Digraphs

Since the auditory dyslexic already has trouble distinguishing between certain consonant sounds, it follows that he will have difficulty with consonant blends. He tends to write the blends with the letters in a transposed order, such as *calm* for *clam* or *paly* for *play* (as does the visual dyslexic, but his reasons are different). As stated before, one must find out how the auditory dyslexic has been taught his phonic elements since learning them in isolation will contribute to these errors.

Sometimes the auditory dyslexic will omit one of the letters of a blend; for example, *mat* for *mast*. And he has special trouble with the *l* and *r* blends (such as in *block, clock, float, glad*, and *bread, crack, drive, frog*).

As for the consonant digraphs (two letter combinations having one sound, such as the *ch* in *chop* or the *th* in *that* or the *wh* in *what*), the auditory dyslexic will come up with just about anything. He often acquires certain mnemonic (memory) devices to help him figure out words. For example, if you listen to him as he reads, you may hear him softly talking to himself as he tries to remember the words. When confronted with *what* he may say, "This word *what* is *at* with a *wh* in front of it," (which it really isn't, of course) or, "*Then* is *hen* with a *t* in front." This is one reason his reading is so very slow and labored and, naturally, this affects his understanding of what he is reading.

Rhyming

Because of his difficulty in distinguishing between words that are similar or different in sound, the auditory dyslexic will not be able to rhyme with any facility, whether he is asked to say words that rhyme or to write words that rhyme with a given word. He does not seem to be able to hear a part of a word and then go through the mental process of relating and associating and supplying words with the same ending. Even high school auditory dyslexics have trouble with rhyming elements.

For example, when asked to say some words that rhyme with *man*, the auditory dyslexic may respond with *mat* or *men*. He may throw in some nonsense words such as *zan, lan*, or *gan*. When asked to write rhyming words, he may just run through the alphabet writing words that rhyme with the key word but which are also gibberish: *ball, call, dall, eall, fall, gall, hall, jall*, and so on. Of course, what he is actually doing is copying the phonogram *all* and then just placing a letter in front of it. The rhyming concept has escaped him. In written rhyming exercises, look for the auditory dyslexic to do this especially if there is an alphabet writing chart in plain sight!

Syllabication

Since the auditory dyslexic has difficulty with auditory analysis and synthesis, he cannot distinguish the different syllables in words. He has problems with dividing words into syllables and with building a word from syllables. Naturally, this disorder affects both reading and spelling. Since he has trouble with syllabication, he has a tendency to omit syllables in both reading and writing, to reverse syllables, and at times to add syllables.

Scrambled Words and Sentences

The auditory dyslexic has trouble accurately retrieving words from his auditory memory. This, together with his difficulty in blending, results in a garbled pronunciation of certain words. Spoonerisms, such as saying "tons of soil" for "sons of toil," are not uncommon. Tongue twisters are very difficult for him to say, even slowly. He really does seem to trip over his own tongue.

While it is common for young children to pronounce *animal* as *aminal* or *spaghetti* as *pasghetti* or *aluminum* as *alunimum* or *enemy* as *emeny*, the older child should be able to articulate these words correctly. But the auditory dyslexic will continue to have trouble with them beyond the normal stage. The letters and syllables of words seem to scramble into different combinations. Too often, at school and at home, people will laugh at and mimic the auditory dyslexic when he comes up with these misarticulations. This may be fun for the others; it is no fun at all for the dyslexic. Unaware of what he has just said, he cannot understand what sets them off. He feels uneasy, self-conscious, and at times defensive.

Parents, brothers and sisters, and teachers need to be sensitive to such mistakes and reactions. They must understand that what is funny to them is embarrassing and humiliating to him. As a defense, the auditory dyslexic may resort to silence—saying as little as possible in front of others—a tragedy, indeed.

Oh, yes, it *is* possible for the auditory dyslexic to learn to laugh along with the others—but only when he feels happy and secure in his environment.

A further point: many of the auditory dyslexics in our clinic have had a history of some early speech disorder that required speech therapy.

Spelling

The spelling errors of the auditory dyslexic result from his difficulty in matching sounds with written words and in retaining the auditory memory of the words. His troubles with vowel sounds, consonant blends, and digraphs have been mentioned. Incorrect vowels will be written, consonant blends broken, letters and syllables added or omitted, and the spelling rules (such as *i* before *e* except after *c*) are meaningless. Words that are similar in sound confuse him. He is just as likely as not to spell *cat* as *kat* or *city* as *sitee*. He cannot reauditorize the rules nor the sounds. He tends to spell "phonetically"—*bot* for *boat, mene* for *many,* or *gos* for *goes.*

He has a great deal of difficulty in acquiring a stock of correct spelling words. His spelling can be more bizarre than that of the visual dyslexic.

"Sarah" came to our reading clinic for help with her reading and spelling problems the summer before she was to enter the sixth grade. She was eleven years old. Testing indicated that she had the mental ability to be able to read at the seventh grade level. However, her instructional reading level was second grade, and her independent or "free reading" level was preprimer. Her instructional spelling level was first grade.

Sarah was very frustrated by her inability to read the assignments in her textbooks and to do the work expected of her in school. She was frank about dreading the arrival of September when she would have to return to school. When asked to write the days of the week in order, Sarah wrote:

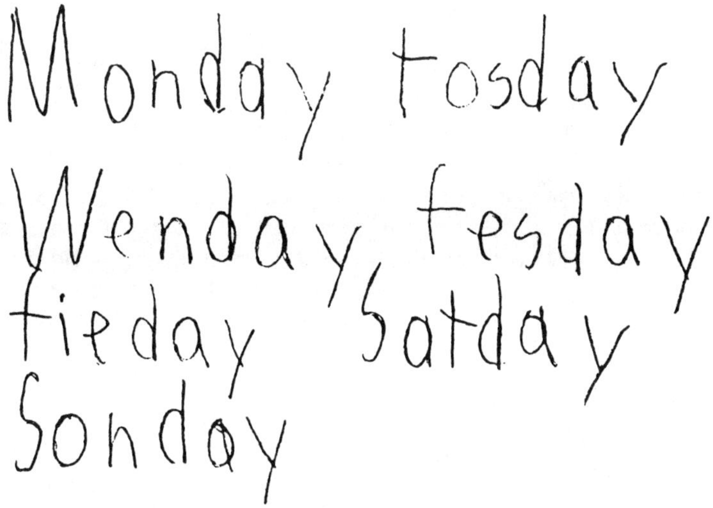

Monday tosday
Wenday tesday
tieday satday
Sonday

Figure 5.3.   The days of the week written by Sarah, an auditory dyslexic. (C.A.11-0,
Gr. 6).

Observe that Sarah wrote the days of the week in correct sequence, even
in a left to right, top to bottom, order. This was not her problem. Note also that
only Monday was spelled correctly, but that she did know how to spell *day* correctly in each word. Her spelling errors consisted of omitting the vowel combination *ue* in Tuesday and substituting the vowel *o*, omitting the *d* and *es* in
Wednesday, omitting the *h* as part of the digraph *th* and the *ur* in Thursday,
substituting the vowel *e*, omitting the *r* in the *fr* blend in Friday, substituting the
vowel *e*, omitting the *ur* in Saturday, and substituting the vowel *o* for the vowel
u in Sunday. These errors are typical of the auditory dyslexic's writing.

Handwriting
The auditory dyslexic writes slowly, but his letter formation is usually
better than the visual dyslexic's. He frequently marks over and erases what he
has written, but this is because of his uncertainty in spelling rather than an inconstancy of letter formation.

Other Subjects in School

As a result of his serious reading and writing disabilities, the auditory dyslexic has difficulties in the other subjects. He cannot read textbooks with understanding. He has trouble attending to lectures and taking notes.

He generally does not enjoy musical recitals and concerts, and has difficulty with the rhythm of music and dancing. He will avoid music classes and band if at all possible. But, to be accepted as "one of the gang," he will often pretend to be "up on the latest," attend rock concerts, and put on a great act.

The dyslexic (whether auditory or visual) often withdraws and becomes an isolate. Or he may take the opposite course and become the "bully" and ring leader of a gang to try to prove his worth to himself and others.

Auditory dyslexics often are good in vocational shop, woodworking, and athletics.

Trying to learn a foreign language can drive an auditory dyslexic to distraction. His auditory processing problems with sound and synthesis make this very difficult for him. Any foreign language requirement should be waved for the auditory dyslexic. He has enough problems with his own language. Learning shorthand or a code, such as the Morse code, presents the same problems of discrimination, association, and processing. The Morse code also requires a sense of rhythm and the use of sound units of dots and dashes.

Standardized Reading Achievement Tests

The auditory dyslexic generally scores higher on the comprehension subtest than on the vocabulary subtest. The words in isolation on the vocabulary test, if unknown, must be figured out by phonics analysis or mental substitution (a form of phonics), or by breaking the word into syllables—all tasks difficult for him—or even configuration (but then several words may have the same shape). The auditory dyslexic is at a loss and is likely to zip through the test, guessing at the answers, marking them at random.

On the comprehension test containing narrative passages, he knows the meaning of some of the words, and he can draw on the context of the story or exercise to figure out others. His visual memory, usually strong, can also help him to locate answers. He will work very slowly, trying to make sense of what he is reading, but as the paragraphs become harder he will probably give up and begin guessing—especially with the pressure of time bearing down on him.

His silent reading score will likely be higher than his oral reading score.

Summary

The auditory dyslexic's major problems are with his ability to integrate and process the sounds of language and to associate them with the written symbols in reading and writing. He has difficulty with reauditorizing what he has heard, and this affects any situation in which listening is involved as well as any in which his own speaking is involved. Every subject in school can be affected by his auditory dyslexia. His dyslexia colors his whole life—home, community, school—and affects his relations with his teachers, classmates, family, and others with whom he comes into contact.

Notes for Chapter 5

1. Stanley W. Jacob, Clarice Ashworth Francone, and Walter J. Lossow, *Structure and Function in Man* (Philadelphia: W. B. Saunders, 1978), pp. 319–325.
2. David D. Caldarelli and Ruth S. Campanella, *The World Book Encyclopedia*, Vol.6 (Chicago: World Book, Inc., 1985), pp. 5–8d.
3. Jacob, Francone, and Lossow, op.cit., pp. 325–326.
4. Doris J. Johnson and Helmer R. Myklebust, *Learning Disabilities, Educational Principles and Practices* (New York: Grune and Stratton, 1967), p. 175.

PART THREE: KEEPING OUR FEET ON THE GROUND

To know just what has to be done, then to do it, comprises the whole philosophy of practical life.

—Sir William Osler

CHAPTER

6

COMMON SENSE AND "EARLY IDENTIFICATION" OF DYSLEXIA

Progress, therefore, is not an accident,
but a necessity.
    —*Herbert Spencer*

Nothing astonishes men so much as common sense and
plain dealing.
    —*Ralph Waldo Emerson*

T he push is on for "early identification" of dyslexia; the rallying cry is, "The sooner we can catch these children the sooner we can begin the remediation of the dyslexia. So let's test as soon as we can to see if we have any dyslexics."

Sounds good, doesn't it? But attempts at identifying dyslexia too early are fraught with problems. The possibility of error carries with it a real danger of premature efforts at remediation which may aggravate a disability or even create one where none existed before. As yet, no test instruments have been devised to identify positively, with validity, those children in nursery school or kindergarten or first or second grades who have dyslexia and those who do not.

Just as it is difficult to distinguish between the young cygnets of the trumpeter swan and those of the whistling swan until the cygnets have matured to a certain degree, so too it is with our young children who may or may not have dyslexia.

At our clinic, a part of the criteria for acceptance is that a child must be at least eight years old or in the third grade. There are reasons for intervention at this age, rather than earlier, that go far beyond any limitations of space, materials, or personnel. These have to do with the child himself—that is, his biological development (maturation), which is gradual and progressive. This is true for all children, although all do not develop at a uniform rate. Children are individuals and they grow as individuals. Each child's maturation and progress in learning are intricately, inevitably intermingled. Some children mature early; others need more time. We refer to what is called the "magical age of eight" in diagnosis for good reasons.

Vision Development

The type is large in primary reading books and gradually decreases with each grade. The reason for this is that most young children are naturally farsighted (hyperopia), but as the child grows, develops, and matures, the eyeball lengthens, and the farsightedness gradually decreases.[1,2] The typical child is about eight years old when his eyes become sufficiently mature to cope with the demands of a school's numerous near-point vision tasks.

When children are farsighted and are asked to do a great deal of close work, the letters and words tend to blur, they become tired, get headaches, and, of course, lose interest in the work at hand. They may become restless and may get into mischief and create problems in the classroom. The teacher is likely to view them as being simply "hyperactive," and "unable to attend to the task" in the pages of the workbook, skill sheets, reading book, or textbook.

Among the various refractive conditions that cause reading disabilities, farsightedness is the most frequently listed. Farsightedness causes both excessive accommodation and convergence.[3] Since many learning disability cases do not have good near-point acuity, most being farsighted,[4] the question may be: might some of these children have been diagnosed as learning disabled (LD) at an early age, before their vision had matured?

There are some educational implications to be considered with regard to children's visual immaturity. Too much close work, too much busy work, too many purple dittoed worksheets, too many workbook pages for young pupils may well be a major factor in contributing to vision problems. Too much close work is being required in too many classrooms, including remedial reading and learning disability classes where young students are frequently deluged by page after page of skill sheets from commercial "cookbook" programs of remediation. It is easy for teachers to use such printed materials to excess.

Early identification? Caution and common sense are needed. As Emerald Decant has pointed out, "Unfortunately, too many teachers fail to recognize the relationship between visual immaturity and failure in reading in the first grade."[5]

Visual Discrimination Development

Visual discrimination is not to be confused with visual acuity—overall vision, the ability to see clearly as determined by vision tests. Visual discrimination is the ability to differentiate between similarities and differences in letters and words, such as between *b* and *d* or *pan* and *pen*. While certain defects in visual acuity may cause some errors in visual discrimination (vision screening should always be a part of diagnostic testing), a child may have excellent vision but poor visual discrimination. Here, too, there are developmental factors to keep in mind when making a diagnosis.

Some authors of articles and books on dyslexia stress the need of assessing dyslexia at the earliest possible moment, and have stated that one of the early identification symptoms to look for is if a child confuses *p* and *b* and *d*, or *no* and *on*, or *horse* and *house*, and the like. As any primary teacher knows, such errors are common among first graders and even second graders. As the students get older and more mature, these types of errors should disappear. It is when such behavior *persists* that we become concerned. Although maturation cannot be hurried, a child's visual discrimination can be sharpened by experience and practice.[6] But care must be taken that this does not involve an excessive amount of near-point work.

Auditory Discrimination Development

Auditory discrimination should not be confused with auditory acuity—overall hearing, the ability to hear sounds of varying pitch and at differing degrees of loudness as measured by a hearing test such as with an audiometer. Auditory discrimination is the ability to differentiate between similarities and differences in speech sounds (phonemes) and combinations of sounds, as in "*big*" and "*dig*," or "*pay*," "*lay*," "*play*," or "pen," "pan," "pin," or "m*a*d" and "m*a*de." Say the following letters aloud and listen to the similarity in sound although each is different:

b, c, d, e, g, p, t, v, z

Some linguists have maintained that if a child can pronounce most words accurately, then he must have adequate auditory discrimination. This would appear to be true; however, the ability to abstract a sound from a spoken word and then compare it with a sound in another word is a cognitive proficiency that many five- and six-year-olds have not yet developed.[7] Those familiar with Piaget's theory of cognitive development will know that this task requires a child to attend to different features and their relationship to the whole word. This is called "decentration."

As with vision, certain kinds of auditory acuity defects (such as a hearing loss of fifteen decibels or high-frequency hearing losses) may cause auditory discrimination errors. A child may have excellent overall hearing but poor auditory discrimination. Maturational factors affect the development of a child's auditory discrimination.

Again, as with visual discrimination, certain authors of articles and books on dyslexia who stress early diagnosis state that problems in auditory discrimination are symptomatic of dyslexia. Yet young children show differing degrees of ability in auditory discrimination; and, furthermore, auditory discrimination rarely is fully developed before the age of eight.[8,9,10] Experienced primary teachers know that most children's auditory discrimination errors disappear as the students grow and mature and gain experience and practice in the classroom, unless, of course, the child has a serious hearing loss.

It is when such auditory discrimination errors persist for no apparent reason that we should become concerned.

Auditory Sequential Memory

Auditory memory difficulties are a part of the syndrome of dyslexia. Again, one should be cautious in applying any such diagnosis to young children. Auditory memory has to do with a child's ability to remember accurately what has been said, whether it is words in isolation or in sentences, or digits in a certain sequence. Auditory memory affects being able to follow oral directions or, indeed, *any* listening task.

The act of reading requires the reader to make the association of a visual sequence of letter symbols (the written word) with an auditory sequence of speech sounds (the spoken word). Writing and spelling require remembering the sequential order of letters that make up a word. The child may transpose letters within words, such as *aminal* for *animal* or *paly* for *play*. Substitutions, omissions, or distortions of words may occur when the child is asked to repeat what he has heard. The young child may pronounce *spaghetti* as *pasghetti* or *enemy* as *emeny*. Any kind of dictation or note-taking exercise is difficult for a child with auditory memory problems.

The ability to recall sequences is developmental in nature. The child gradually becomes able to recall longer and longer series of words, sentences, or digits. Usually there is little change in scores on various tests of auditory sequential memory between the ages of seven and eight. The most significant changes occur between the ages of six and seven[11]—that is, generally students in the first and second grades.

Visual Memory

Visual memory refers to the ability to remember letters, words, objects, and events seen. A strong visual memory is essential for learning and remembering those words in our language to which the phonics rules do not apply (irregular words), such as *head, break, once, does, through, though,* or *rough*.

A child will never read fluently until he has acquired a stock of sight words—words that the reader must recognize instantly without interrupting his reading. Visual memory is necessary for acquiring a necessary stock of words. It is also needed to learn handwriting and to remember how each letter is shaped. Intelligence is considered to be a related factor, although it is possible for a very bright child to have poor visual memory.

The maturity of a child's development in vision and visual discrimination plays an important role in visual memory.

Spelling

A strong visual memory is far more important than phonics for accurate spelling. Spelling is basically a matter of convention and etymology. It is the meaning of the words that provides clues to the spelling of many words. For words that contain "silent" letters, such as in *heat* or *light*, and the irregular words, the child must draw upon his visual memory. He must "see" (revisualize) the *gh* in *light* because those letters are not heard. He must remember that these letters are in the word so as not to spell the word as *lite*. He must keep a *visual image* that *one* is not spelled *won*, the way it sounds.

Spelling errors are often analyzed and used in the diagnosis of dyslexia. This practice with very young students is highly questionable in view of the various stages of spelling which children go through. As children are growing and gaining experiences, they seem to construct tentative rules based on their knowledge of the language, and then they apply the rules to their spelling. Primary teachers know well how *yor* eventually becomes *yours*, how *tod* becomes *tode* and then *toad*, and *lafwts* becomes *elefant* and finally *elephant*. A child's visual memory plays a part in this evolution of accuracy in spelling. Recent studies have established that there is a sequence of spelling stages through which children go, and their knowledge about written words is acquired in a systematic, developmental, and gradual manner.[12,13]

Dyslexics cannot be placed neatly and cleanly within the developmental spelling stages. It is as though their spelling progress had been arrested at points along the way, with ups and downs in a rather erratic pattern of progress. Both visual and auditory dyslexics can have bizarre misspellings, although auditory dyslexics tend to have more.

Too early attempts at identification of dyslexia on the basis of errors in spelling may result in misdiagnosis, with serious implications for the child. There are *normal* types of errors that children make as they progress through the developmental spelling stages, each child in his individual manner. All do not make exactly the same errors.

These types of spelling errors must not be misconstrued as dyslexia symptoms in the young child. Later, if such errors persist in the older child, appropriate steps for referral should be taken.

Visual-Motor (Eye-Hand) Coordination

Visual-motor coordination refers to the ability of a child's eyes and hands to work together in such tasks as writing, copying, cutting with scissors, pasting, coloring, tying shoelaces, buttoning coats, stringing beads, using hammers, and throwing or catching or batting a ball. These tasks may be required when testing a child for hand preference. Writing a story and copying from a chart are two tasks required in the dyslexia diagnostic battery.

Gross motor skills are developed before the finer motor skills. The latter are required for the tasks mentioned above. For this reason, children are usually first introduced to the manuscript ("printing") style of writing. The straight lines, circles, and spacing forms are much simpler for the young child than the more complex movements required for cursive writing. Most authorities believe that until about the third grade—or about the age of eight—many children do not acquire the intricate muscular development and maturity needed to learn cursive writing.[14,15,16]

Experience based on various experiments indicates that cursive writing can be learned in the third grade, after two years of manuscript writing, more easily than in the first or second grades, and the quality of writing in the upper grades is equal to or superior to the writing of children who begin cursive in the first grade.[17]

Children tend to write more if they are permitted to continue using manuscript in the primary grades. They use a greater variety of words and more running words. Indeed, one study[18] of third grade students indicated that each half-year delay in teaching cursive writing increases the mastery of the written language:

— 2,623 different words were used by those who had changed to cursive writing in the second grade,
— 3,798 different words were used by those who had changed in the first half of the third grade,
— 4,636 different words were used by those who had changed in the second half of the third grade, and
— 7,681 different words were used by those who had continued using manuscript writing throughout the third grade.

The Bender Visual-Motor Gestalt Test used by some in "detecting" dyslexia requires the child to copy certain designs containing curved and straight lines, dots, little circles, and open and closed figures, with the forms becoming increasingly more complex. Of interest here is that the Bender test score tends *to improve during the primary grades*[19]—that is, as the child matures, and as he develops his fine motor control. Any difficulty may not at all be due to the child's inaccurate perception of the figures. Actually, the reliability of the

Bender test with young school children is poor, and test-retest scores vary considerably, especially during the first two school years.[20]

Visual-motor coordination seems to reach maturity somewhere between age six and age eight.[21] Since the finer muscle development of most little boys lags behind that of most little girls, the majority of boys will take longer to acquire the maturity for such coordination.

Lateral Awareness/Directional Confusion

Lateral awareness refers to a child's ability to discriminate right from left, and difficulty with this is often regarded as being one of the symptoms of dyslexia. But young children are often confused when a teacher gives directions involving the use of the words *right* and *left*. When they do not follow these directions they are considered disobedient. A child may be told to get the book on the right side of the bookcase, and then when he stands there in confusion, he may be scolded for not doing what he has been told to do. Such experiences occur at home as well as at school. Children may have trouble in physical education classes for the same reason.

By the age of seven, a child may have developed an awareness of the right and left parts of his *own* body (left eye, right foot) which is sometimes referred to as "personal space awareness." Most children are able to do this by age eight, but some are not until age nine, and mental age has an influence upon the performance level. However, the lateral awareness for such tasks, as in the example above—where the teacher gave directions regarding the bookcase, called "extra-personal space awareness"—is not established until children are between the ages of nine and twelve years.[22,23] Note that a range of ages is given, not one certain age where this occurs for *all* children.

Problems in personal space awareness and extra-personal space awareness are usually considered symptomatic of dyslexia, and tests for such difficulties are included in the dyslexia diagnostic battery. But parents and teachers (and diagnosticians) must keep in mind that there are developmental aspects in acquiring this lateral awareness. The maturity of the child must be taken into account before any final decision can be made as to whether a child is dyslexic.

Language Acquisition

Young students are still learning to speak distinctly and to produce sounds correctly. There is a relationship between hearing and auditory discrimination with speech development. Of course a hearing loss can affect the development of speech in a child. So too, while a child may have a keen sense of *hearing*, problems with being able auditorily to discriminate between the various sounds can contribute to difficulties in speech. But beyond this, many normal children in the beginning years of school cannot articulate certain sounds well. Young children make frequent common substitution errors which follow a pattern. It is not unusual for young students age six to age eight to substitute the following sounds: [24]

/f/ for /v/, and sometimes /v/ for /f/
/f/ for the /th/ sound heard in *thin*
/s/ for /z/
/k/ for /t/
/n/ for /m/
/th/ as heard in *thin* for the /th/ as heard in *that* and also for /s/

Young students seem to have particular problems in pronouncing /r/, /l/, and /s/, and these sounds (phonemes) make up the major articulation therapy loads of public school speech therapists.[25,26] It follows that primary grade children have special trouble with the *r, l,* and *s* blends, such as *tr, dr, cr . . . bl, cl, fl . . . sc, sk, sl . . .* and so on.[27]

Young students have more difficulty producing certain sounds in the middle of words and at the end of words than they do at the beginning. Growth and maturation, however, eliminate many articulation errors in the first few grades.

The pattern of speech development has implications for any phonics assessment since auditory discrimination is linked to speech development. Some teachers try to teach certain phonic elements to children who cannot even pronounce those elements accurately, much less discriminate between those sounds.

Authors of articles and books on dyslexia often mention that confusing the sounds mentioned above, as well as making errors in the middle and end of words, is symptomatic of dyslexia. It would be very easy to come up with a misdiagnosis of dyslexia if one should test children at too young a developmental age.

There are certain developmental shifts in children's acquisition of language. These shifts concern not only the speech sounds and changes of sounds, but also the patterns of words in sentences and the meanings of words and how these meanings can change. These are referred to as the phonological, syntactical, and semantical shifts in a child's language development.

The periods between the ages of five and eight and then again between the ages of twelve and fourteen are marked by instability in linguistic development. These are then followed by growth and stable linguistic performance. During these two periods there are large increases in the child's new grammatical constructions and high error rates in some kinds of these constructions.[28, 29]

These age ranges concur with Piaget's cognitive development transition points, when the child moves from preoperational thought to concrete operations (age five to eight) and from concrete operations to formal operations (age eleven or twelve and up).[30] The concrete stage is the first stage of operational intelligence, and it is here that the child begins to classify and group things—ideas—and to understand numbers and things in series, but he needs real (concrete) objects in order to learn and to apply these concepts. Formal operations involve considering various alternatives of a situation, making propositions, understanding proportions in mathematics, and solving problems on the basis of logic.

Language development and cognitive development are intimately interwoven, intricately related, with developmental patterns that must be taken into account when one is planning instruction or diagnosing dyslexia.

Finger Agnosia/Finger Localization

Finger agnosia refers to the relative, or absolute, inability to indicate which fingers, or how many, have been touched by an examiner. Children who have finger agnosia tend to have poor handwriting with inconsistent letter formation and size. In both spelling and reading they will transpose letters within words, such as *clam* for *calm*. They erase frequently and tend to have many strike-overs of letters. And their handwriting rate is slow, so that such children often cannot finish their work in the time allotted. Students with this problem are likely to do poorly on drawing tests, such as the Bender-Gestalt Test or the Slosson Drawing Coordination Test, thus confounding the findings.

Finger localization shows a progressive development beginning about the age of four; by age eight or nine most tasks can be performed by the average child. The localization of stimulated single fingers on a tactual basis alone shows rapid development through years seven to nine. By the age of nine, performance is about 93 percent correct as compared with 67 percent by age six. Performance in the localization of single fingers on a tactual-visual basis is 98 percent by age eight, as compared with 88 percent by age six. Mental age has a strong influence on performance.[31]

A child can have finger agnosia and not be dyslexic. Yet all too frequently children with finger agnosia are misdiagnosed as being dyslexic because their writing and spelling errors are similar to those of the dyslexic. This test is sometimes administered to children at too early an age for any valid conclusions to be drawn from the results.

Myelination within the Brain

Nerve cells in our brains contain a nucleus and a long fiber, or projection, of varying length (along which the nerve impulse travels) called the *axon*, and a diverse but extensive number of branching fibers of varying length called *dendrites* that reach outward toward other nerve cells. There is a fatty

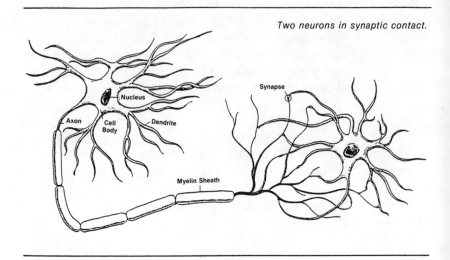

Figure 6.1   Myelin sheath encasing the axon. (From *The Brain*, by Richard M. Restak, New York: Bantam, © 1984, p. 27.)

substance which covers the axon, called the *myelin sheath*. (Figure 6.1.) A nerve impulse is carried along the length of the axon, where it ends on various numbers of dendrites or cell bodies of other nerve cells.

What is important to our discussion on early identification of dyslexia is that the process of myelination of a nerve axon is not completed until late childhood.[32] This type of maturation in the brain is said to have implications in teaching abstract concepts and certainly could affect the validity of early identification of dyslexia in very young students.

Some Other Matters to Consider in Diagnosing Dyslexia

There are other matters that need to be taken into account, and to which common sense should be applied, when considering any early identification of problems in young students. A child just simply may not care for the whole idea of school and would far prefer to stay home. He may have a "personality conflict" with his teacher and have no desire to please her, particularly with progress in schoolwork. It is possible too that he may have hostile feelings toward his parents who pressure him to read—and so he won't. And then, it is conceivable that a child just may not understand at the time what reading and writing are all about, and thus may not be at all interested in learning, in which case more time is needed for barriers to be overcome and for the business of learning to get under way.

Reading Readiness Tests

What about reading readiness tests? Don't they examine some of the very factors which have been discussed in this chapter?

Of course they do. They can be used to *help* a teacher decide if a particular child is ready to be moved into formal reading instruction. A reading readiness test, along with a checklist of behavior and achievement in various areas based on observations, and probably some type of mental maturity test, can make a useful contribution to the teacher's experienced judgment.

But the results of a reading readiness test should never be used alone to make a decision for formal reading instruction. They are by no means infallible. The range of positive correlation with school achievement is from .40 to .70 for most major reading readiness tests. This may be fairly substantial for a whole group but it is of little value in predicting the achievement of an individual student. Clearly, the prediction for success (or lack of success) in reading does not hold for a large percentage of the children taking the test. In any case, readiness for reading cannot be equated with the actual reading process. Reading readiness serves as a foundation for and a bridge *into* reading.

Reading readiness tests may reveal certain areas of weakness as well as strengths to help the teacher in planning certain activities, but a child is not just a collection of various skills. (Nor is reading.) The *whole* child is involved in learning. Reading readiness tests and other types of developmental tests do *not* specify which students are dyslexic and which are not.

Summary

Early attempts at identification of dyslexia—prior to the age of eight—are ill-advised. Many of the symptoms of dyslexia are related to the normal developmental growth of the child, mentally and physically, so the possibility of misdiagnosis is great. Unfortunately, such misdiagnoses are being made. Misdiagnoses not only harm children but also create a great credibility gap when such findings are examined by experts in child growth and development who are aware of the relationship of maturation to reading, writing, and spelling. This, no doubt, has contributed to the present confusion about dyslexia.

Insofar as possible, the developmental factors contributing to dyslexia-like symptoms must be ruled out first. For example, at the present time there is no valid way to determine whether the reversal of *b* and *d* in a six or seven year old is due to the level of development of visual discrimination and spatial perception or to dyslexia.

It *is* possible, of course, to determine if a vision defect is contributing to certain problems. It should be possible to discover if a child has been taught the phonic elements in isolation, thus viewing the *d*, *i*, and *g* in the word *dig* as three separate elements rather than viewing the word as an entity and tend ing to reverse either the *d* or *g*.

The instruction of a child must be considered in any diagnosis as a possible cause of certain types of errors similar to those of dyslexia. The school curriculum must be considered from the standpoint of whether a child has had the opportunity to learn certain information. For example, the days of the week and the months of the year are usually part of the dyslexia test battery. One must ask: is a child unable to say these in sequence because he is dyslexic, or simply because he has not yet had an opportunity to *learn* them in school? Common sense must be applied in any such situation.

When the dyslexic pattern of errors persists and the child gets older and moves through the grades, then our concern is with a correct diagnosis followed as soon as possible by a program of remediation designed to alleviate the various difficulties which result from this very real disability.

Notes for Chapter 6

1. Emerald Dechant, *Diagnosis and Remediation of Reading Disabilities* (Englewood Cliffs, N.J.: Prentice-Hall, 1981), p. 164.
2. Albert J. Harris and Edward R. Sipay, *How to Increase Reading Ability*, 7th ed. revised (New York: Longman, 1980), p. 28.
3. Eldon E. Ekwall, *Diagnosis and Remediation of the Disabled Reader* (Boston: Allyn and Bacon, 1976), p. 198.
4. George Kaluger and Clifford J. Kolson, *Reading and Learning Disabilities* (Columbus, Ohio: Charles E. Merrill, 1978), p. 128.
5. Dechant, op.cit., p. 164.
6. Arthur W. Heilman, Timothy R. Blair, and William H. Rupley, *Principles and Practices of Teaching Reading*, 5th ed. (Columbus, Ohio: Charles E. Merrill, 1981), p. 104.
7. Harris and Sipay, op.cit., p. 26.
8. Dainis Turaids, Joseph M. Wepman, and Anne Morency, "A Perceptual Test Battery: Development and Standardization," *Elementary School Journal* 72 (1972), p. 352.
9. Anne Morency, "Auditory Modality and Reading, Research and Practice," *Perception and Reading*, Helen K. Smith, ed., Vol. 12, Part 4 (Newark, Delaware: International Reading Association, 1968), p. 18.
10. Dechant, op.cit., p. 250.
11. Ibid., p. 252.
12. James W. Beers, "Developmental Strategies of Spelling Competence in Primary School Children," *Developmental and Cognitive Aspects of Learning to Spell: A Reflection of Word Knowledge*, Edmund H. Henderson and James W. Beers, eds. (Newark, Delaware: International Reading Association, 1980), pp. 36–45.
13. J. Richard Gentry, "An Analysis of Developmental Spelling in GNYS AT WRK," *The Reading Teacher* 36 (November 1982), pp. 192–200; "Learn to Spell Developmentally," *The Reading Teacher* 34 (January 1981), pp. 378–381.

14. Paul C. Burns and Betty L. Broman, *The Language Arts in Childhood Education* (Chicago: Rand McNally College, 1979), pp. 330, 338.
15. Gertrude A. Boyd, *Teaching Communication Skills in the Elementary School* (New York: Van Nostrand Reinhold, 1970), p. 44.
16. Virgil E. Herrick, "Children's Experiences in Writing," Virgil E. Herrick and Leland B. Jacobs, eds. (Englewood Cliffs, N.J.: Prentice-Hall, 1955), pp. 271–272.
17. Boyd, op.cit., p. 44.
18. Louis Ada Wilson, "A Study of Some Influencing Factors Upon and the Nature of Young Children's Written Language," *Journal of Experimental Education* 31 (1963), p. 374.
19. Albert J. Harris and Edward R. Sipay, *How to Teach Reading* (New York: Longman, 1979), p. 42. Also: Edwards, Alley, and Snider in an investigation found no evidence that a diagnosis of minimal brain dysfunction based on a pediatric neurological evaluation and/or visual-motor impairment as measured by the *Bender-Gestalt* is a useful predictor of academic achievement. The investigators deem that a multi-disciplinary approach is necessary in the diagnosis of learning problems. R. Phillips Edwards, Gordon R. Alley, and William Snider, "Academic Achievement and Minimal Brain Dysfunction," *Journal of Learning Disabilities* 4 (March 1971), pp. 17, 20.
20. Elizabeth M. Koppitz, *The Bender Gestalt Test for Young Children* (New York: Grune and Stratton, 1971), pp. 38–39. Also: Spache states, "If the Bender gave some diagnostic information for the teacher . . . there might be some justification for its use in readiness testing. But in view of its unreliability and lack of constructive interpretation I could not recommend it." George D. Spache, *Diagnosing and Correcting Reading Disabilities*, 2nd ed. (Boston: Allyn and Bacon, 1981), p. 38.
21. Dechant, op.cit., p. 256.
22. Arthur L. Benton, "Right-Left Discrimination," *Pediatric Clinics of North America* 15 (1968), p. 753; *Right-Left Discrimination and Finger Localization, Development and Pathology* (New York: Harper and Brothers, 1959), pp. 27, 36.
23. Spache, op.cit., p. 44.
24. Katherine Snow, "A Comparative Study of Sound Substitutions Used by 'Normal' First Grade Children," *Speech Monographs* 31 (1964), pp. 138, 141.
25. Mildred C. Templin, "The Study of Articulation and Language Development During the Early School Years," *The Genesis of Language, A Psycholinguistic Approach* Frank Smith and George A. Miller, eds. (Cambridge, Mass.: The MIT Press, 1966), pp. 176–177.
26. Alvin M. Liberman, "General Discussion: Temple Presentation," *The Genesis of Language, A Psycholinguistic Approach*, Frank Smith and George A. Miller, eds. (Cambridge, Mass.: The MIT Press, 1966), p. 183.
27. Boyd, op.cit., p. 110.
28. David S. Palermo and Dennis L. Molfese, "Language Acquisition From Age Five Onward," *Psychological Bulletin* 78 (December 1972), p. 422. Also: The left side of the angular gyrus (inferior parietal lobule in the brain) is critical for receptive language and is the last cortical area to reach full cellular development, often not until late childhood. Paul Satz and Sara S. Sparrow,

"Specific Developmental Dyslexia: A Theoretical Formulation," *Specific Reading Disability, Advances in Theory and Method*, Dirk J. Bakker and Paul Satz, eds. (The Netherlands: Rotterdam University Press, 1970), p. 25.

29. Paula Menyuk, "Middle and Late Childhood," *Language and Maturation* (Cambridge, Mass.: The MIT Press, 1977), pp. 89–122.

30. Jean Piaget, " The Stages of the Intellectual Development of the Child," *Readings in Child Development and Personality*, Paul Henry Mussen, John J. Conger, and Jerome Kagan, eds. (New York: Harper and Row, 1970, 1965), pp. 296–197.

31. Benton, (1959), op.cit., pp. 67–69, 145.

32. Drake D. Duane, "A Neurologic Overview of Specific Language Disability for the Non-Neurologist," *Bulletin of the Orton Society* 25 (1974), p. 15.

CHAPTER

7

FIVE CHILDREN: DYSLEXIC OR NOT?

There are no unteachable children.
There are only schools and teachers and
parents who fail to teach them.

—Mortimer J. Adler

No bubble is so iridescent or floats
longer than that blown by the
successful teacher.

—Sir William Osler

In order to illustrate the hazard of attempting to diagnose serious problems in young students, I have summarized the reading achievements of five children as they progressed through kindergarten and the early elementary grades. All of these children were of average or high average intelligence. Their profiles indicate their individual patterns and will help in understanding why an early "diagnosis" of dyslexia is perilous.

Mary

Mary's growth in reading was steady throughout her early school years. Her progress record is typical of many children. She was a stable, self-confident child, somewhat large for her age. With her birthday in February, she was not a "young" kindergarten child when she began school. In fact, she was almost a year older than some of the children in her class. She was popular with her classmates and teacher and often was chosen as a leader in group activities. She enjoyed story and reading time, and when she was in kindergarten and first grade she would pick up picture books and sit quietly looking at them. As she acquired independent reading skills, she began reading books on her own whenever she could. Fortunately, she was in a school where the principal's priority was for "the teachers to have the tools to do the job," and so each classroom had a variety of books at different levels for the students to use for their free reading time, for which time was set aside each day in addition to the time a child might have after finishing the assigned work.

As Mary moved up through the grades, her teachers reported that her enjoyment of reading served as a motivation for her to finish her seatwork as quickly as she could so as to have additional time for reading.

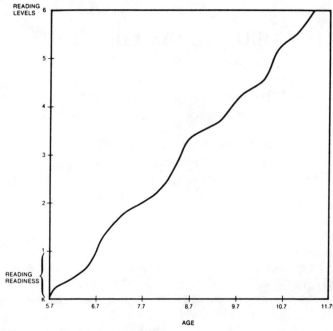

Figure 7.1   Mary's progress in reading.

Mary liked to write stories. She quickly mastered manuscript writing and began writing short stories of her own which she would illustrate. Her writing was well-formed and was soon reduced in size, and she began writing on one line instead of two. She probably could have learned cursive easily in the second grade, but she was in a school system where cursive writing was introduced in the third grade. At that time her teacher, who individualized handwriting instruction, decided that Mary could begin instruction right away. Mary then learned cursive writing very quickly, and her writing was excellent.

From the beginning her spelling showed good progress. Her visual memory was strong, and she retained the irregular spellings of words with little difficulty.

When administered the reading readiness test at the beginning of first grade, Mary's scores in all areas were high. The prediction then, based on testing and observations, was that she would achieve successfully in reading. This she did, as indicated by her reading achievement progress profile on page 88.

Tommy

Tommy was a little live wire, full of energy, curious, not the least bit interested in sitting at his desk and doing his seatwork. Fortunately for Tommy, his kindergarten teacher believed that this was a time for children to continue to grow and develop in all areas, not just academic skills. Periods of inactivity and sitting quietly were interspersed with periods of action and movement,

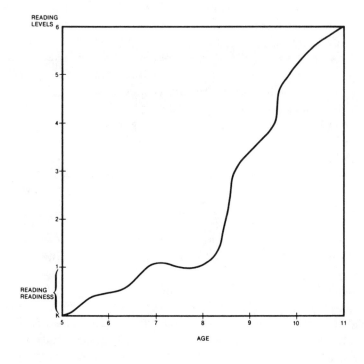

Figure 7.2   Tommy's progress in reading.

singing and dancing, acting out stories, finger painting, working with clay, pretending to be animals or butterflies or trains or whatever.

Readiness groups were set up after the Christmas holidays, and by the end of the year a couple of the children were beginning to read. A reading readiness test was given at the end of kindergarten, and Tommy's scores were somewhat low. In the fall, after several weeks of school, Tommy's first grade teacher gave the reading readiness test again to use as a diagnostic instrument to give her some direction as to his areas of weakness and strength. His scores were just about the same as in kindergarten.

He had some reversal problems, confusing b with d, and p with q. The possibility of dyslexia did not enter the teacher's mind. Again Tommy was fortunate, for his teacher understood that he was somewhat immature for his age. (He was a June birthday child.) She gave him work that he could do at his level of achievement.

The teacher set up groups within her class according to the different children's needs. At first all were in various readiness groups, but six children were soon moved into a formalized reading group and began their practical charts and preprimers. The teacher used experience charts with all groups and for many different activities. Tommy was happy in first grade. It did not bother him that he was only at the primer level by the end of the school year. It did bother his parents who thought that Tommy would do better with a teacher who "used more structure" than those Tommy had had in kindergarten and first grade. They asked the principal to place Tommy in Mrs. X's class the following year because she had the reputation of being a strict disciplinarian.

Tommy's second grade year was disastrous. His teacher arranged the chairs in rows rather than in nests of tables because "this kept children out of mischief and their hands to themselves." She had only three reading groups, Tommy being in the lowest. While she worked with one group, the other children had workbook pages and dittoed seatwork sheets "to keep them busy and quiet," and when this was done there was always work to copy off the chalkboard.

Tommy never got to the chalkboard work; he rarely finished his seatwork, and every day he had to take the incomplete work home with him to finish after school. He resented having to stay in afternoons when he wanted to climb the big tree in his yard and work on the tree house with his buddy. He resented losing the "privilege" of swimming with a "bunch of the guys" at a nearby indoor pool each Saturday because he always had all that unfinished schoolwork to do. His parents told him that when he began doing his work at school as he was supposed to, he could do these other things. And his mother reported that she resented having to sit with him every afternoon when he got home from school to see that the work got done, as well as after dinner when she had to bathe the baby, get her to bed, and get the supper dishes washed.

What happened to Tommy? He became balky and moody, both at school and at home. He was not a happy child. His scores took a nose dive. He was still confusing *b* with *d* and would often write the capital *B* for the lower case, as in *BaBy*. The teacher suggested to his parents that this was a symptom of dyslexia which Tommy probably had, and she went on to say that there was nothing much that could be done for children like that. She recommended that Tommy repeat the second grade.

The parents, in turn, talked with the principal and explained Tommy's problems in class. The principal did not say much other than that perhaps Miss Jones should be his third grade teacher. Since the parents were not very happy about the possibility of Tommy repeating the second grade, they agreed to this arrangement.

Third grade was a completely different story. Miss Jones was a bubbly, enthusiastic, creative teacher, full of energy. It was obvious that she enjoyed being with children and teaching. After a few weeks of various activities— games for reviewing vocabulary words and skills, easy reading books for some children and picture books for others, with lots of experience chart stories (and always a positive attitude with Tommy and the other children) and keeping them busy in ways other than with workbooks and dittoed skill sheets— Miss Jones administered several tests so as to set up various groups in her classroom according to the individual needs of the children.

She called Tommy's parents in for a conference and tactfully suggested that they "back off a bit" and lessen the pressure on Tommy. She shared the information she had obtained from her testing and explained what she intended to do to help Tommy. The parents returned home, encouraged about Tommy's school situation, still worried somewhat but optimistic about his third-grade year with Miss Jones.

Within a very short time, Tommy's attitude and performance showed a dramatic change. His progress soared steadily, and it continued to rise. By the end of the third grade he was reading at the third-grade, first-semester level— a big jump from the preprimer to which he had sunk in the second grade. As shown by Tommy's progress chart on page 89, by the end of the fourth grade Tommy was just moving into the fifth-grade level.

Suppose Tommy had been diagnosed as being dyslexic on the basis of his low kindergarten scores or first-grade scores as part of some school early identification program. Was his slow start due to developmental factors, or to dyslexia? Was his drop in achievement in the second grade due to dyslexia as his teacher suggested, or to his school experiences, his relationship with his teacher, her teaching style, and the quality of instruction?

Of course Tommy was not dyslexic, or he could never have made such rapid progress in the third grade and thereafter. And it is probable that had his second grade been in a different classroom things would have fallen into place sooner and his achievements would have been even higher in the later grades.

Sue

Sue was a September birthday child. Her progress was a bit slow until third grade when she began performing on grade level. Then her progress speeded up so that by the time she was ten years old and in the fifth grade she was reading over a year above grade level.

Her profile shows plateaus amidst her rising progress in reading. Such

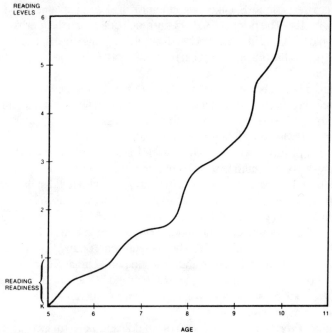

Figure 7.3   Sue's progress in reading.

plateaus are typical in children's learning. In Sue's case, she got off to a slow start, achieving mediocre to low scores on the reading readiness test; but, given time to mature, with nurture and understanding, encouragement and quality instruction, she took off and progressed steadily. Her progress was as shown above.

Had Sue been mistakenly identified as a dyslexic or a child with learning disabilities on the basis of her slow start and test scores, her story might well have been different. Luckily for Sue, she was in a school where the principal and teachers understood the developmental factors that may temporarily affect early progress in school. They were ready to give her special help if she did not begin to improve, but no intervention became necessary.

Larry

Larry was born in November, and thus was a young child in kindergarten. Some of his classmates were almost a year older. He was small for his age and the youngest child in his family. It was especially difficult for his mother to let go of this, her last little chick, and Larry sensed her reluctance. The first few weeks of kindergarten were rough for all: child, teacher, parent. Eventually, the transition was made, and the tears ended.

Larry's scores were low on the various developmental tests and on the reading readiness test administered at the conclusion of kindergarten. They were still low when the test was again administered a few weeks after first grade began. The predictions were that he would likely continue to have problems and that his progress would be slow. Larry's parents were greatly concerned and had frequent conferences with his teachers and the principal. They kept insisting that more special testing be done, and toward the end of the first grade this was arranged. The school evaluation team consisted of his classroom teacher, school psychologist, learning disabilities teacher, a Title I reading teacher, and a special education supervisor. It was agreed that Larry showed many of the symptoms associated with dyslexia. And this was the diagnosis.

The next year Larry began going to a special learning class for an hour three times a week. He was not happy doing this, and told his parents that "there are a bunch of dummies in there and I'm *not* a dummy!" He also told his parents that all they did was work on phonics skill sheets in workbooks. He was happy, however, with his second-grade teacher who planned special work for him at his level, encouraged him to act out stories he had heard or read, and gave him much positive encouragement. Toward the end of the second grade she was sure that he was beginning to make progress at a faster rate. She suggested to his parents that they contact a reading specialist acquaintance of hers and make arrangements to have him tutored over the summer on a regular basis. She also cautioned them to avoid pressuring him and to let him enjoy the summer activities attractive to a boy his age.

Larry hit it off right away with the reading specialist, who was quite creative, had a variety of concrete and interesting materials to use, and provided challenging and exciting reading, spelling, and writing experiences for each session.

Larry's chart shows the startling change in his rate of achievement. At the beginning of third grade, at the recommendation of the tutor and the parents, Larry was not put in any special classes. The parents did request the reading specialist to continue to work with him one afternoon a week on a private basis. This she did for about six months. By fourth grade, Larry was reading comfortably at grade level, as can be seen by the progress below:

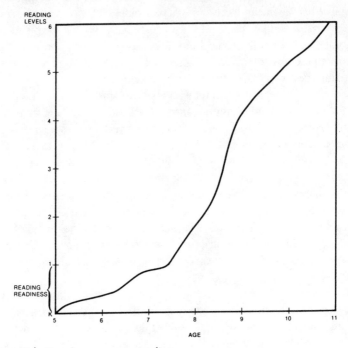

Figure 7.4   Larry's progress in reading.

Larry had been diagnosed as being dyslexic because of his poor performance in early testing. Had he been tested at age eight, no such diagnosis would have been made.

Bruce

Bruce's chart is similar to Larry's in kindergarten and the early grades, except that Bruce repeated the second grade. Unlike Larry, Bruce did not begin to show rapid progress, but continued in his poor achievement.

Bruce came to the clinic when he was ten years old, reading on a first-grade level. An analysis of the total test findings and observations revealed that Bruce did have dyslexia.

An examination of Bruce's school records indicated that at first Bruce was considered just immature. As time went on his parents were told that he could do the work if he weren't so lazy, but that he also needed more growing up time. He was retained in second grade because of his low reading achievement, but he was also having serious problems in arithmetic. All this was very upsetting to Bruce who knew that he was having trouble and was not doing the same level of work as most of his classmates, but he could not understand why he could not move to the next grade with his friends. (Later, in the clinic, he told me that he used to go home after school and crawl under his bed and cry, holding an old blanket against his face to muffle any sound.)

Progress in second grade the second time around showed no improvement. It was as though he sat in class each day and nothing happened, accord-

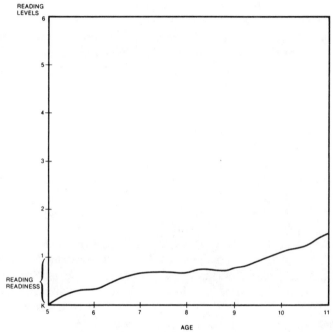

Figure 7.5   Bruce's progress in reading

ing to the end-of-the-year achievement test scores. The school did not want to retain him again at the lower level, and he was promoted to the third grade where his teacher took a special interest in him. She sensed something was really wrong. She "didn't know what, but there was something there I couldn't put my finger on." She knew that Bruce was intellectually capable of learning because she had the results of a special school psychological testing. Bruce made a little progress during his year with her, but very little.

In January, his teacher called his parents and asked that they come in for a conference. At that time she recommended that they contact me for possible diagnostic testing. Bruce attended school some forty miles away, and for various reasons no testing could be done until the following summer when his parents enrolled him in our summer clinic.

Bruce's mother and father were deeply concerned about him. They had continued in their support of Bruce, and had done some of the things many parents do in such cases. They had gone along with the school for a while, then blamed the first grade teacher (she "didn't push phonics" hard enough), proceeded to have his vision and hearing checked by medical doctors, and visited a psychologist for mental tests and to discover why his attitude was so bad and why he would not work at school.

Bruce began wetting his bed, and his parents decided on their own that the pressure of everything was just too much for him. They stopped the visits to the psychologist, whose office was about fifty miles from their home and caused a major logistics problem since both parents were working. There was no change either for the better or the worse, except in the summer Bruce stopped wetting his bed.

Being kept back in school had upset Bruce so much that he refused to play any more with two of his neighborhood friends, who had been in his class but had moved on to third grade when Bruce stayed back. Up to this time, in spite of his problems in school, Bruce had always been popular with the children in both his class and his neighborhood, and he had been something of a leader, sometimes into mischief. He was a good swimmer and had been on the swimming team at the neighborhood swimming pool. Now he began to shun activities and to become something of a loner.

Bruce was feeling that sense of failure, frustration, and loss of self-esteem so common to children with his difficulty and experiences. In this case we would have liked to have begun work with him a year earlier, before such feelings had taken a toll, yet after the required time for the maturational pattern to unfold. For Bruce, intervention came at a good enough time to help him with his problem, and before he had developed that hard shell of protection and facade frequently acquired by dyslexics as a coping device, and which often fools others into thinking the young student means it when he says he doesn't really care—about learning, about school, about anything.

This is nonsense, of course, for children like Bruce *do care*—very much.

CHAPTER
8

THE HISTORICAL DEVELOPMENT OF THE CONCEPT OF DYSLEXIA

Progress, therefore, is not an accident, but
a necessity.

—*Herbert Spencer*

The concept of dyslexia has its roots in two other types of disorders. One is alexia, which refers to a condition in persons who were previously literate but have lost their ability to read as a result of an acquired disease of or injury to the central nervous system. Alexia (note the prefix "a" which means "without") is thus different from dyslexia, which refers to the disability which *prevents* the child from normally acquiring the developmental reading skills. Alexics at one time *could* read. The other type of disorder is aphasia, which is the loss of speech.

Some Early Connections

The early findings that showed that the ability to read might be impaired by brain damage have led to many current investigations of the neurological abnormalities in children with severe reading, writing, and spelling difficulties. In 1834 Professor Lordat of Montpelier, France, who had recovered from a speech disorder in 1825, described his previous inability to make sense of the printed word.[1] He could hear and understand words, but had lost his ability to read. He wrote:

> The alphabet alone was left me, but the function of the letters for the formation of words was a study yet to be made. When I wished to glance over the book which I was reading before my malady overcame me, I found it impossible to read the title. I shall not speak to you of my despair, you can imagine it. I had to spell out slowly most of the words, and I can tell you by the way how much I realized the absurdity of the spelling of our language. After several weeks of profound sadness and resignation, I discovered whilst looking from a distance at the back of one of the volumes in my library, that I was reading accurately the title *Hippocratis Opera*. This discovery caused me to shed tears of joy.[2]

Lordat's story had a happy ending, for his loss of the ability to read was temporary. The point here is that this problem occurred in connection with a speech disorder. As time went on other physicians described instances of patients who had aphasia and became unable to read.

In 1872 Sir William H. Broadbent,[3] Physician to and Joint Lecturer on Medicine at St. Mary's Hospital, London, described a case to the Medical and Chirurgical Society where a man suffered an acute cerebral attack after which he was unable to read printed or written words, except his own name. The patient, Charles D., wrote correctly from dictation and wrote letters with a little prompting, but could not read what he had written. He conversed intelligently, using an extensive vocabulary, but occasionally forgot names, streets, persons, and objects. He was unable to name his arms or legs or the colors of things. The man died soon afterwards from another vascular attack. An autopsy revealed one new and two old lesions ("clots") in his brain. Broadbent believed that one of the older lesions caused the reading difficulty because of its specific location in the man's brain, the left angular (and supramarginal) gyrus. Figure 8.1 shows the location of the angular gyrus in the brain as well as the location of other areas specifically involved in the language process.

In this case the patient could speak and pronounce words correctly and could write from dictation, but he could not recall certain names nor could he read.

In 1877 a German physician, Adolph Kussmaul, coined the term "word-blindness." He noted that while the ability to read could be lost, vision, the power of speech, and the intellect might remain.[4]

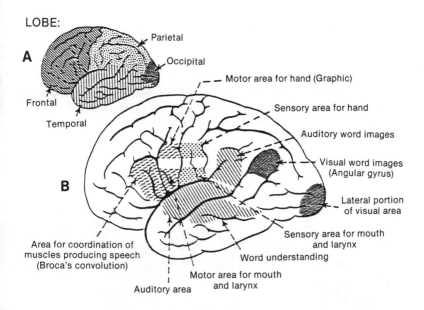

Figure 8.1.   (A) Lobes of the surface of the left hemisphere of the brain, and (B) the hemispheric sites involved in the language processes. (From "A Neurologic Overview of Specific Language Disability for the Non-Neurologist," by Drake D. Duane in *Bulletin of the Orton Society*, 24, 1974, p. 13. Used with permission.)

Kussmall (and Broadbent) were among the first to point out that word-blindness could be dealt with clinically as an isolated condition, and that it represented the pathological condition of a special faculty.[5]

In 1877, Dr. Rudolph Berlin of Germany coined the term, dyslexia (Dyslexie) as an alternative to word-blindness. Berlin had collected six case histories over a period of twenty-three years. In each case, the patients' manner of reading was the same. Each could read the first three to five words, but could read no more. Their speech remained fully intact.[6]

Dyslexia—Congenital?

The suggestion that dyslexia might be a congenital (constitutional) problem probably began with the reports of the doctors James Hinshelwood, W. Pringle Morgan, and James Kerr.

Dr. Hinshelwood[7] was an opthamologist in Glasgow, Scotland. He was surgeon to the Glasgow Eye Infirmary and assistant to the professor of Clinical

Medicine in the University of Glasgow. Over a number of years, various persons had come to him because of their sudden loss of the ability to read, and they thought that the problem might be the result of a vision defect, which was not the case. The patients had lost their reading ability after "fits" or strokes or periods of extreme mental worry.

From 1895 on, Dr. Hinshelwood wrote a series of papers for *The Lancet* about these alexics. He noted that (1) some could recognize the individual letters of the alphabet but not words, (2) some could read a few words and then no more (similar to Dr. Berlin's patients), (3) some could recognize neither letters nor words but could recognize Arabic numerals, and (4) some could read words but not letters. Among these, some patients tended to lose their way in familiar surroundings.

Then, in 1900, within two months of one another, two boys, ages ten and eleven, were brought to Dr. Hinshelwood because the medical attendants where they were examined suspected that their difficulty in learning to read might be due to some cerebral problem. These boys were intelligent but were having an extremely hard time in school. Hinshelwood observed that their symptoms and problems with reading were similar to those that appeared in adults who had suffered brain injuries and lost their ability to read. He also noted that there were often several cases of such reading problems in one family. Hinshelwood noted further that these two cases were excellent examples of different degrees of "congenital word-blindness" in which there were congenital deficiencies in visual memory for words and letters. And he also reported on two other congenital word-blind cases that he had read about in an article by Dr. W. Pringle Morgan, whom Hinshelwood credited with reporting the first case of congenital word-blindness.

Dr. Morgan was a general practitioner who lived in the small town of Seaford in Sussex, in the southern part of England. He had become acquainted with a fourteen-year-old boy, Percy F., who was the oldest son of an intelligent family. In 1896, Morgan wrote a report for the *British Medical Journal* in which he described some of Percy's problems. Morgan had read Dr. Hinshelwood's article on word-blindness and visual memory published in *The Lancet* in 1895 concerning adults with alexia. Morgan could find no reference anywhere to the possibility that the condition was congenital, and yet Percy F. had had trouble learning to read from his earliest schooling. Morgan stated that Percy's condition followed "upon no injury or illness" and was "evidently congenital, and due most probably to defective development of that region of the brain, disease of which in adults produces practically the same symptoms—that is, the left angular gyrus." [8] (See Figure 8.1.) Morgan wrote:

> His great difficulty has been—and is now—his inability to learn to read. This inability is so markable, and so pronounced, that I have no doubt it is due to some congenital defect . . .

The following is the result of an examination I made a short time since. He knows all his letters and can write them and read them. In writing from dictation he comes to grief over any but the simplest words. For instance, I dictated the following sentence: "Now, you watch me while I spin it." He wrote: "Now you word me wale I spin it"; and again, "Carefully winding the string round the peg" was written: "Calfuly winder the sturng rond the Pag."

In writing his own name he made a mistake, putting "Precy" for "Percy," and he did not notice the mistake until his attention was called to it more than once . . .

I then asked him to read me a sentence out of an easy child's book without spelling the words. The result was curious. He did not read a single word correctly, with the exception of "and," "the," "of," "that," etc.; the other words seemed to be quite unknown to him, and he could not even make an attempt to pronounce them . . .

He seems to have no power of preserving and storing up the visual impression produced by words—hence the words, though seen, have no significance for him. His visual memory for words is defective or absent; which is equivalent to saying that he is what Kassmaul has termed "word blind." . . .

I may add that the boy is bright and of average intelligence in conversation . . . his eyesight is good. The schoolmaster who has taught him for some years says that he would be the smartest lad in the school if the instruction were entirely oral.[9]

A short time later, in 1897, Dr. James Kerr, a school medical officer of Bradford, in the Midlands of England, wrote a school hygiene essay in which he called attention to mentally intelligent children with problems similar to Percy F.'s who were extreme cases needing consideration by the school and teachers.[10]

Dr. Hinshelwood continued to collect data on such cases, which were now referred to as "congenital word-blindness," and he published another book on the subject in 1917. Others began reporting similar observations over the following years, with the result that "word-blindness" in those early days was suspected as due to either cerebral damage or a congenital defect in children with normal or undamaged brains.

In the United States a neuropsychiatrist, Samuel T. Orton, had been observing some children with reading and writing problems who reversed letters and seemed to find it easier to write from right to left. He coined a new term, "strephosymbolia" (from the Greek), which literally means the turning or twisting of symbols. Dr. Orton believed that these difficulties were due to an abnormality of brain function, a confusion in the memory images of symbols. Like Hinshelwood, Orton considered that the problem was congenital. Orton, however, suggested that strephosymbolia was caused by the genetically determined failure of one brain hemisphere to assume the dominant role in mediating language and speech functions.[11] But his theory has never gained general acceptance because the patterns of reading, writing, and spelling mistakes of dyslexic children cannot be adequately explained in terms of such confused mirror images, and also because of the difficulty in testing the neurological propositions.[12,13,14] (Dr. Orton's theory is explained in more detail in the next chapter.)

Nevertheless, Dr. Orton is considered an American pioneer in dyslexia, and an organization dedicated to helping children with dyslexia and other learning disabilities has been named after him. His work and that of his disciples aroused interest in children who had severe problems in learning to read, with the result that papers about such children began appearing in the United States as well as in European countries.

Help on the Way

Help for the dyslexic child was on its way although it would be some time before it would become effective. The deluge of papers, studies, and reports—some clear, some ambiguous; some objective, some biased; some valid, some not; some in agreement, some contradictory; some professional, some amateurish—contributed to the growing knowledge, yet also succeeded in muddying the waters of research and providing ammunition for the skeptics.

Notes for Chapter 8

1. Macdonald Critchley, *The Dyslexic Child* (Springfield, Illinois: Charles C. Thomas, 1970), p. 1.
2. Ibid.
3. Sir William Henry Broadbent, "On the Cerebral Mechanism of Speech and Thought," *Medico-Chirurgical Transactions*, The Royal Medical and Chirurgical Society of London, Vol. 37 (London: Longman, Green, Reader, and Dyer, 1872), pp. 162–165.
4. Sandhya Naidoo, *Specific Dyslexia, The Research Report of the ICAA Word Blind Center for Dyslexic Children* (New York: John Wiley & Sons, 1972), p. 2. As time passed, more and more autopsies were performed and lesions, softenings, or hemorrhages in the occipito-parietal region of the left cerebral hemisphere were found in some of these persons. The occipital lobe and the parietal lobe are in the cortical areas behind the central fissure. (The latter is the slight furrow which runs downward from the top over the outer portion of the hemispheres, and with the longitudinal sulcus, a deep ditch running front to back, and the Sylvian fissure along the outer side of each hemisphere at about the level of the angle of the jaw—divide the cerebral hemispheres into artificially separate territories.)

5. James Hinshelwood, *Congenital Word-Blindness* (London: H. K. Lewis, 1917), p. 1.

6. Rudolph F. Wagner, "Rudolf Berlin: Originator of the Term Dyslexia," *Bulletin of the Orton Society* 23 (1973), pp. 60–61.

7. James Hinshelwood, "Word-blindness and Visual Memory," *The Lancet* (Dec. 21, 1895), pp. 1564–1570; "A Case of Dyslexia: A Peculiar Form of Word-Blindness," *The Lancet* (Nov. 21, 1896), pp. 1451–1454; "A Case of 'Word' Without 'Letter' Blindness," *The Lancet* (Feb. 12, 1898), pp. 422–425; " 'Letter' Without 'Word' Blindness," *The Lancet* (Jan. 14, 1899), pp. 85–86; "Congenital Word-Blindness," *The Lancet* (May 26, 1900), pp. 1506–1508; *Congenital Word-Blindness* (London: H. K. Lewis, 1917), p. 77.

8. W. Pringle Morgan, "A Case of Congenital Word Blindness," *British Medical Journal* (Nov. 7, 1896), p. 1378.

9. Morgan, op.cit., p. 1378.

10. James Kerr, "School Hygiene, in its Mental, Moral, and Physical Aspects," *Journal of the Royal Statistical Society* Vol. 60, (1897), p. 668.

11. Samuel T. Orton, " 'Word-blindness' in School Children," *Archives of Neurology and Psychiatry* 14, No. 5 (November 1925), p. 610; *Reading, Writing, and Speech Problems in Children* (New York: W. W. Norton, 1937), pp. 68–118.

12. Donald G. Doehring, *Patterns of Impairment in Specific Reading Disability, A Neuropsychological Investigation* (Bloomington: Indiana University Press, 1968), p. 8.

13. M. D. Vernon, *Backwardness in Reading, A Study of its Nature and Origin* (Cambridge: Cambridge University, 1958), pp. 82–110.

14. Calvin Tomkins, "The Last Skill Acquired," *New Yorker* Vol. 39 (Sept. 14, 1963), p. 146.

15. Naidoo, op.cit., p. 8.

CHAPTER

9

WHAT CAUSES DYSLEXIA?

Somebody said that it couldn't be done,
But he with a chuckle replied,
That "maybe it couldn't," but he would
be one
Who wouldn't say so till he'd tried.

—*Edgar Guest*

W hat causes dyslexia? Have the neurosurgeons, general medical practitioners, psychiatrists, geneticists, developmental experts, education specialists, or school psychologists finally found any answers over all these years? The answer is: maybe partially. Knowledge is accumulating. But until diagnoses become more accurate, criteria of research more clearly established, reports of findings more carefully drawn, and until explorations of the functioning of the brain are more complete, and objectivity replaces concern for pet theories, no final answers can be expected.

The search must continue. In spite of all the barriers erected by those whose major interests lie elsewhere, in spite of all the criticisms of ill-informed skeptics, in spite of all the frustrations of working with contradictory reports and incomplete information, the search must continue for the sake of those who do have dyslexia. We can, in fact, diagnose dyslexia accurately, but accurate diagnosis does not necessarily imply any definitive answer as to the cause.

Common sense and high standards of professionalism must prevail in all cases. Undoubtedly, a major factor in extravagant claims concerning a "cure" for dyslexia is due to a misdiagnosis in the first place. For example, one person (a psychiatrist) claims to have cured "thousands" of dyslexics over the last ten years. He has attracted a good deal of attention in the media with the assertion that he has found THE cause of dyslexia, and the cure is drugs and vitamins. However, upon reading his books, one finds that some of his "dyslexics" were excellent readers and spellers. (One excellent speller was a *proofreader*!) True, his children patients were having problems in school and at home, such as poor attitudes, dislike of schoolwork or school, inconsistency in work performance, headaches, stomach-aches, moodiness, emotional problems, hyperactivity, and so forth. He even made the statement that *all* of his "phobic patients were found to have dyslexia."

At the present time, just what have we investigated? Why does dyslexia occur in a small percentage of the population? What is the progress to date?

Is Dyslexia Inherited?

Research on the question of whether genetics has anything to do with dyslexia has consisted mainly in studies on the concordance (both twins having dyslexia) of identical (single-ovum/monozygotic) twins and the concordance of nonidentical (dizygotic) twins, or family history and pedigree analysis.

Studies of twins have been sparse, but the concordance has been 100 percent for identical twins and about 33 percent for nonidentical twins. Information on Hermann's[1] summary of studies of forty-five sets of twins and Zerbin-Rubin's[2] summary of ten studies of fifty-three sets of twins is given in Appendix B for the reader who wishes to investigate these further.

What about the families of dyslexics? Is there a tendency in other members of the family to have similar disabilities? A pedigree chart can illustrate the affected and unaffected brothers, sisters, parents, and other relatives of dyslexics and the distribution of dyslexia (if any) in families. One should be aware of certain problems in making such a pedigree analysis with regard to the occurrence of dyslexia in several successive generations. In the case of the grandparents of the dyslexic child, it may be difficult to make a diagnosis of dyslexia because the researcher may not be able to get the satisfactory historical data. Even if one or more of the grandparents did have dyslexia, the condition may have been relatively mild and could have been unobserved for various reasons at that time. It is also possible that a dyslexic adult may deny that he has dyslexia for one reason or another.

Figure 9.1 is a pedigree chart for which data were obtainable on the grandparents. The following symbols and abbreviations are used:

Squares designate males.

Circles designate females.

Solid black indicates dyslexia.

One slash indicates a person who was too young for diagnosis or who died before reaching the "age of manifestation."

Crossed lines indicate data were lacking for an accurate diagnosis of dyslexia.

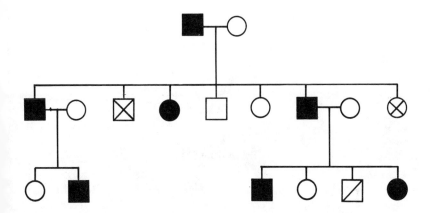

Figure 9.1. Pedigree chart of dyslexia for three generations.

As can be seen by the chart, the grandfather was dyslexic; the grandmother was not. They had seven children of whom two sons and one daughter were dyslexic. A son and daughter were definitely not dyslexic, but the conditions of another son and daughter could not be determined because of insufficient data. One dyslexic son married a nonaffected woman, and they had two children, a dyslexic son and a daughter who was not dyslexic. Another dyslexic son married a nonaffected woman and they had four children, two of whom were dyslexic, one daughter who was not, and one son who was too young for a diagnosis of dyslexia to be made. Dyslexia is known to have occurred in three generations in this case.

Figure 9.2 is a pedigree chart prepared by Hallgren.[3] The dyslexic child was sent to him by his colleagues, and he was able to trace dyslexia for four generations. He reported that the majority of the members of this family were very talented, and their intellectual capacity was high. Nonetheless, dyslexia caused definite difficulties at school and later in life for family members who did have the condition. The numbers 1, 2, 3, and 4 on the chart show the four

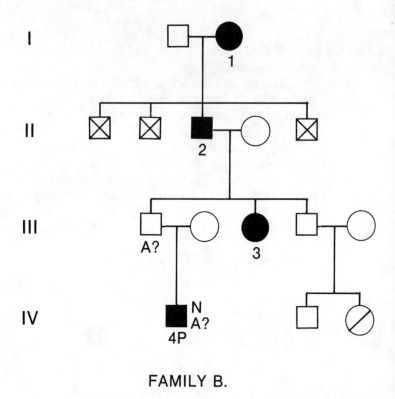

FAMILY B.

Figure 9.2. Hallgren's pedigree chart showing four generations of dyslexics. (From *Specific Dyslexia* ("*Congenital Word-Blindness*"); *A Clinical and Genetic Study,* by Bertil Hallgren, Copenhagen: Ejnar Munksgaard, © 1950, translation from the Swedish by Erica Odelberg, Stockholm: Esselte aktiebolag, 1950, p. 274. Used with permission.)

generations of dyslexics. Members with *A?* have suspected specific arithmetical disability. The letter *N* by the youngest dyslexic indicates that he is a "problem child."

Since the above family was "selected," Hallgren did not include it in his genetic-statistical analysis of dyslexia in 112 families. Here he found that in ninety families, one parent had dyslexia. In three families, both parents had dyslexia. In nineteen families, neither parent was dyslexic. Direct inheritance in three generations was found in twenty families. In four of these families, two or more affected members in the direct line belonging to the same generation had dyslexia.[4]

Other family history studies have revealed the following information:

Study 1:   40 percent of the parents had reading problems, while less than 10 percent of the parents of nondyslexic children had reading problems.[5]

Study 2: 39.7 percent of the dyslexics had one or more close relatives with related learning problems.[6]

Study 3: 36.7 percent of the families of dyslexics had problems, with 22.5 percent for those of a control group.[7]

Study 4: In sixteen families with a child having "specific reading disability," in which both parents were tested and classified, three dyslexics had both parents affected, ten had only one parent affected. Three children had neither parent affected.[8]

Is dyslexia inherited? Findings such as these would indicate that certainly in some cases dyslexia is genetically determined, that it does seem to "run" in some families. But while there appears to be a genetic aspect to dyslexia, the linkage has not yet been definitely established. Various hypotheses have been made, studies are continuing, but nothing has been conclusively proved.

Maturational Lag

Is maturational lag the cause of dyslexia? A maturational lag is the slow or delayed development of those brain areas that bring about the acquisition of certain developmental skills which are basically age-linked. In Chapter Six, concerning the early identification of dyslexia, I explained the developmental factors that can affect achievement in certain school tasks. These maturational factors were spelled out in terms of the typical child's development, and it was pointed out that some children develop earlier, some later, but within a certain range of age, usually by age eight—but sometimes later for some children in some areas—most children have acquired the required maturity. A maturational lag implies cerebral immaturity.

It is true that some children get off to a slow start in school, and as time passes, some of these "late bloomers" begin to sail along and catch up. The question is: are these children really dyslexic, or is their individual developmental pattern only somewhat deviant from that of the "typical" child? Some children just need more time to get moving; others take off right away and progress faster. The child who learns to read later may become a better reader than one who begins earlier.

Children do not progress in a lock-step fashion, all together and at the same time. They are *individuals* and progress in an individual manner, although the *overall pattern* may be similar. Their individual perceptual boundaries change with age because of the structural and functional alterations in their general growth processes, and the consequent decentration of perception.[9] Levels and rates of maturation may vary a great deal among *normal* children.

Much of the discussion on maturation lag as a cause of dyslexia rests on pure speculation. The research studies have been done mainly with kindergarten, first grade, and second grade children, with a few at other levels. What were the findings of such studies? Some children were more advanced in

certain perceptual skills (such as visual discrimination and auditory discrimination) and knowledge; others less so. Surely this was not unexpected. Any
kindergarten or primary grade teacher knows that some children start off
slowly, test poorly, and then after a few weeks or months, things seem to "jell"
and they move up. In other words, poor readers may develop into good readers. Of course, some young children perform poorly and continue to do so.
Unfortunately, in many of the studies no mention of intelligence is made—a
factor that can certainly affect a child's academic progress, and a variable that
should be taken into account in any such study.

It is possible that there may be some kind of maturation lag for a number of children as a result of cerebral immaturity, but could this not happen to
children who are *not* dyslexic as well as to those who are? This may be a partial
explanation for those "late bloomers." And *if* maturation lag were the cause of
dyslexia, then it would follow that there would be three different kinds of
"lags"—one that causes visual dyslexia, another that causes auditory dyslexia,
and still another that causes a mixture of visual and auditory dyslexia.

*If this really were the basic cause, would not dyslexics naturally "grow
out" of the condition in time?*

The notion that maturational lag causes dyslexia remains just that at the
present time—a notion based on speculation only. It is highly improbable that
any *tangible* evidence will emerge any time soon.

Cerebral Dominance (Lateral Dominance)

The brain is divided into two hemispheres, the left hemisphere controlling the right side of the body, and the right controlling the left side of the
body. (See Figure 9.3.)

Consistency in the use of one side of the body to dominate motor functions (right-eyed, right-handed, right-footed, or vice versa) is usually considered as evidence of neural integrity in the central nervous system. But many
people do not have this clear-cut dominance. Some are left-eyed, right-
handed, and right-footed (or right-eyed, left-handed, and right-footed, or any
other variety of combinations). This is called mixed or crossed dominance.

Some dyslexics have crossed dominance; some do not. Some superior
readers and spellers have crossed dominance; some do not. About 90 percent
of the population are right-handed, with 10 percent left-handed, but approximately 60 percent of the left-handers process speech in the left hemisphere
just as right-handed persons do. The other 40 percent of the left-handers appear to use both sides.[10]

There is a fine, but important distinction between the terms *ambidex-
terity* and *ambivalency* in the use of the hands. An ambidextrous person is able
to use both hands equally well for some tasks, and may do this even though
one hand is considered the dominant, or preferred hand. But ambivalency (in
the technical sense used here) implies a conflicting use in the hands, using

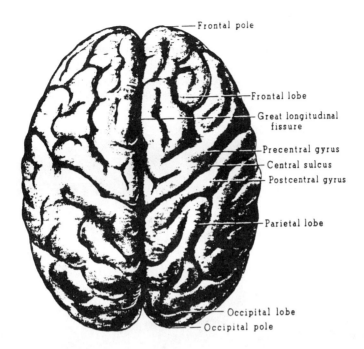

Figure 9.3.   Superior view of the two hemispheres of the brain. (From *Structure and Function in Man*, by Stanley W. Jacob, Clarice Ashworth Francone, and Walter J. Lossow, Philadelphia: W. B. Saunders, © 1982, p. 242. Used with permission.)

either about half the time, with no dominant (preferred) hand, and is sometimes referred to as unestablished dominance. Some researchers have found a correlation of ambivalency in the use of hands with reading, writing, and spelling problems (not necessarily dyslexia).

Dr. Samuel Orton suggested in 1925 that strephosymbolia (dyslexia) was caused by confusion between the two hemispheres of the brain. He believed that memory images in the right hemisphere are the exact mirrored counterpart of those in the left hemisphere. For example, if the word *not* were stored in the left hemisphere, it would be stored as *ton* in the right hemisphere. If *saw* were stored in the left hemisphere, its mirrored counterpart in the right hemisphere would be *was*. He believed this was the reason for the twisted symbols and reversals of dyslexics.[11]

Figure 9.4 illustrates Orton's theory of mirrored images in the two hemispheres. Note that the letters *ABC* in the left hemisphere are shown in reversed form in the right hemisphere.

By 1937, Orton was suggesting that the confusion of the two brain hemispheres was caused by mixed or crossed dominance. Although Orton's views are no longer accepted, the notion that mixed or crossed dominance is the cause of reading difficulty or dyslexia still persists among some educators.

Occasionally, one hears in the classroom the comment, "Oh, he has reading problems. He has mixed dominance, you know."

Research never has established that mixed or crossed dominance causes dyslexia or any other type of reading disability.

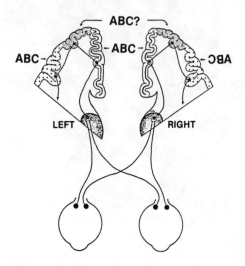

Figure 9.4. Orton's theory of memory images in the left hemisphere having mirrored counterpart images in the right hemisphere. (From " 'Word-blindness' in School Children," by Samuel T. Orton, *Archives of Neurology and Psychiatry*, November 1925, 14, p. 609. © 1925, American Medical Association. Used with permission.)

Neurological Dysfunction

In the preceding chapter on the historical development of the concept of dyslexia, the term *alexia* was explained as a condition in which persons who were previously literate had lost their ability to read as a result of acquired disease of or injury to the central nervous system. The term in general use today is *acquired dyslexia*. Research is both scarce and rather mixed on acquired dyslexia. Reference to control groups in the literature is rather sparse, even though control groups are essential to establish whether certain errors in reading and spelling are due to an improper reading and spelling development (stages, etc.), or to dyslexia.

Another term the reader will encounter is *developmental dyslexia*, which implies no brain damage. Yet various doctors have suggested that the dyslexic's difficulties may be neurological in origin. Parents can become greatly upset by such terms as "minimal brain dysfunction" and the like. Unfortunately, some educators have become confused, and they view dyslexia as a medical condition. As a result, in some schools improper screening procedures are used to identify children with learning problems. For example, in preschool screening, some school personnel make indefensible assumptions about motor development and certain types of neurological difficulty affecting reading, writing, and spelling achievement in school. As a consequence, some schools have set up "motor development programs" where children walk beams, jump through old tires, throw balls and bean bags, draw big circles, and go through other similar activities with the idea that this will make the children better readers and spellers.[12] The connection has not been made. Probably all this will do nothing but improve the children's balance, throwing, and drawing, and give them a little fun and exercise.

It has also been suggested that dyslexia could be caused by certain prenatal difficulties or birth complications such as anoxia (lack of sufficient oxygen), but research so far has not established this linkage. Certain diseases and high fever affecting the child's brain may be a cause, but there is no solid proof of this either.

Dyslexia and the Use of the EEG

The validity of the electroencephalogram (EEG) to indicate different modes of brain pathology has been established for years. But the usefulness of the EEG with dyslexics has been disputable, and the controversy continues. Some dyslexics have "abnormal" EEG findings; some do not. Some superior readers and spellers have "abnormal" EEG findings; some do not.

How does the EEG work? Pieces of metal which act as conductors (electrodes) are placed on different parts of a person's scalp. These electrodes pick up the brain waves transmitted from the part of the brain nearest to the electrode. These waves are passed into a machine where they are amplified and then traced onto moving graph paper. The neurologist examines these patterns to determine if the brain is functioning normally. For example, the presence of slow waves in the occipital region, or positive spike patterns, or epileptiform discharges are characteristic of abnormal EEGs.

There have been numerous studies made, but no EEG pattern has been established as a correlate of dyslexia; that is, there is no proved relation between the two. For example, in a study of eighty-two dyslexic children, where detailed information was obtained from families, maternity hospitals, nurseries, nursery schools, regular schools, attending doctors and hospitals, it was found that on neurological investigation, *the most severe degree of dyslexia could exist without any evidence of brain damage.*[13]

In fact, G. Keith Connors reviewed a number of studies and concluded that they could just as easily be "interpreted as showing the *absence* of EEG abnormalities among dyslexics," and that the better-controlled studies especially lead to this interpretation.[14] (A list of various problems that Connors encountered with studies is included in the Notes for this chapter.)

The notion that there is some general, unspecified neurological abnormality causing dyslexia has not been proved.

Beyond the EEG with the BEAM and SPM

Brain electrical activity mapping (BEAM) is a way of adding to the amount of information obtained on a standard EEG. When the neurologist reads the EEG, he analyzes the brain waves recorded on the graph paper. The BEAM does not create new data, but converts the squiggly lines of the EEG into a color-coded map. The results can be compared to what happens when a column of numbers is converted into color graphics. The information already there becomes more apparent.[15] (See Figure 9.5.)

The significance probability mapping (SPM) depends upon a computer-driven statistical analysis that shows, point by point, whether a particular EEG pattern deviates from the normal pattern. Dr. Richard M. Restak[16] neurologist, reports that both "BEAM and SPM are already proving highly reliable in clinical diagnosis. BEAM and SPM are correct 80 to 90 percent of the time when diagnosing dyslexia in ten-to-twelve-year-olds. Brain tumors can also be detected by BEAM with an accuracy at least 10 percent better than relying on standard EEGs."

No information was given regarding this diagnosis of dyslexia in ten to twelve year olds other than that cited. I would like to know *how* this was determined, what *knowledge* was acquired, what *criteria* were used. Did follow-up testing of their reading, spelling, and writing problems affirm the accuracy of the diagnosis? Were the children *first* diagnosed by other means and afterwards given the BEAM and SPM as a check? Or vice versa? If the use of the EEG with dyslexics is disputable, then, *since the BEAM and SPM interpretations are based on the EEG, should not the validity of these results be questioned?*

An increase of 10 percent in detecting brain tumors is an improvement and certainly to be desired, but this is quite different from *diagnosing dyslexia*. I already know how to diagnose dyslexia—but what about the *cause* of dyslexia? Were any insights as to its causation obtained? This is what we are searching for.

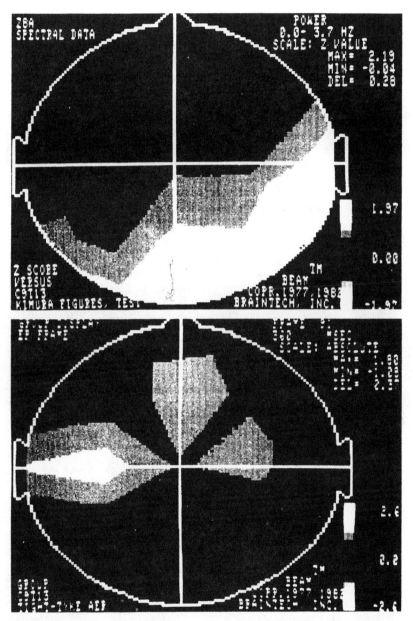

BEAM scans can be combined into a single scan for study. Top, lighter areas indicate where brain electrical activity in dyslexics dif- fers most from that in a group of normal readers; below, the control group

Figure 9.5.   (From *The Brain*, by Richard M. Restak, New York: Bantam, © 1984, p. 243.)

Specialization Within the Brain

As already mentioned, the brain is divided into two hemispheres. At one time there were two conflicting views. The traditional view held that the two hemispheres of the brain were simply mirror images of each other (Orton's view, for example), with no reason to designate particular functions to one hemisphere rather than to the other. The other view was that the hemispheres were specialized, and some things are done better by one or the other hemisphere. The latter view has come to be accepted. The left hemisphere is concerned mainly with language, verbal reasoning, and certain motor skills, while the right hemisphere is more adept at certain kinds of spatial functions, such as understanding and working with maps, visualizing and remembering faces, and other performances that do not depend on verbal descriptions.

We now know, however, that the functions of one hemisphere, though specialized, are not necessarily exclusive. A number of exceptions recently has led neuroscientists to re-evaluate their thinking about specialization within the brain. Further experiments have indicated that the brain just does not break down, as has previously been suggested, into neat little categories—each hemisphere with its own functions altogether exclusive of the other hemisphere.

With the discovery of the PET Scanner (Positron Emission Tomography) which currently is being used to "map" the brain, new knowledge is being uncovered about the functions of the hemispheres. Hemispheric specialization has been found to occur along *different* lines in *different* people.[17]

Music awareness has been considered a right hemisphere function. In a "landmark experiment" at the University of California at Los Angeles, research scientists have compared PET scans of persons listening to music after having been given certain directions. The scientists discovered that the brain responds differently depending upon the cognitive strategies which the listener uses! An example task: two musical chords were sounded and the person was asked if the chords were the same ones or different. If the person just listened and answered reflexively (perhaps by pushing one button if the chords were alike or another if they were different), the right hemisphere of the brain was likely to carry out the task, thus responding according to perceptions. But if the person responded by mentally arranging the chords along the piano keys, drawing on visual memory and imagery, then the task shifted to the more symbolic mode of the left hemisphere.[18] What is important here is the cognitive strategy used by the listener and the fact that *either* hemisphere could be used.

Other research has expanded our understanding of the functions of the brain hemispheres. Rather than saying that the left hemisphere is specialized for language, the more accurate phrasing would probably be that the left hemisphere is specialized for symbolic representation; whereas the right hemisphere deals more with representations that reflect reality more directly—that is, those chunks of experience that do not use language. To make it clearer and to avoid oversimplifications, one might say that the brain is divided into the *symbolic-conceptual hemisphere* (left) and the *nonsymbolic directly-perceived hemisphere* (right).

But it is not exactly true that the right hemisphere is wholly lacking in language ability, for it can decode words such as "dog" or "house," after some practice, although it may have trouble with symbolic words such as "liberty" or "honesty." It seems, in any case, as if the right hemisphere can get meaning more easily from concrete objects and events.[19]

It appears also that we need *both* hemispheres for language, although the left is considered the more important of the two for this function. Why? An injury in "Broca's area" (in the *left* hemisphere; see Figure 9.6) can cause a person to be unable to say a simple straightforward sentence, such as, "Is this what you really wanted?"

Recent research at the Texas Health Center in Dallas and also at Harvard University has shown that disorders in the *right* hemisphere can cause a per-

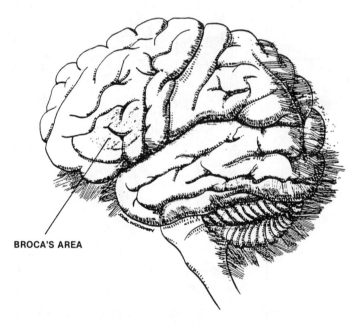

BROCA'S AREA

Figure 9.6.   "Broca's area" is vital to speech and language ability. (From *The Brain*, by Richard M. Restak, New York: Bantam, © 1984, p. 238.)

son to lose the capacity to distinguish the *important nuances* of everyday speech, such as subtle shades of meaning, emotional tones of sarcasm, disbelief, or irony. It is as though the right hemisphere furnishes us with the emotional aspects of our speech—the color, the liveliness, the spirit. For example, an injury to our right hemisphere could make it impossible to intone some subtle irony if the above sentence were said in this way, "Is THAT what you really wanted?" Our words would ring flat.

There is no doubt that both sides of our brain are needed. In fact, along with Restak, one can say with "equal validity that we are not just the right and left sides of our brain but simply we are our brain."[20]

What does specialization within the brain have to do with dyslexia? We

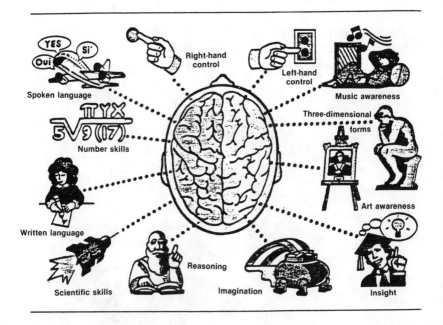

Figure 9.7. The multifaceted brain. (From *The Brain*, by Richard M. Restak, New York: Bantam, © 1984, p. 260.)

need the information to set the foundation to increase our understanding of dyslexia for it brings up some interesting questions. While neurological dysfunction has not been proved to be a cause of dyslexia, to date, most of the dyslexia research appears to have viewed the two hemispheres as having separate functions. But surely the recent discoveries concerning the cross-over and inter-relationship of the two hemispheres suggest that further thinking along this line is needed. Some researchers[21] even speak in terms of "R-type dyslexics" (excessive development of right-hemispheric reading strategies) and "L-type dyslexics" (excessive development of left-hemispheric reading strategies).

Should not this "either-or" mentality be altered to consider the inter-relationship of both hemispheres? What about the different hemispheres used in responses by different persons? Do these new findings not have implications for the remediation of dyslexia?

Obviously, we need to know more about the workings of the brains of dyslexics. We need to get *inside* the brains to determine what answers may lie there. The opportunity to examine a brain occurs frequently, but the chance to examine the brain of a diagnosed dyslexic is very, very rare.

The Brain of a Dyslexic

In 1979, a twenty-year-old male "dyslexic" died of multiple internal injuries as a result of an accidental fall from a great height. His brain had not been directly injured in this fatal accident. Dr. Albert M. Galaburda and Dr. Thomas L. Kemper[22] from the Departments of Neurology, Harvard Medical School and Boston University School of Medicine, and the Neurological Units, Beth Israel Hospital and Boston City Hospital, received permission to examine the young man's brain.

The young man's difficulties with reading and spelling caused him to repeat the first grade and the diagnosis of dyslexia was made at that time, during which a routine neurological evaluation indicated no abnormal findings.

He was the youngest of four children, three boys and one girl. His father and both of his brothers were slow readers, but not his mother nor his sister. He, and several other family members, were left-handed. He received special tutoring but continued to have trouble with the language arts. Table 9.1 shows his reading achievement test scores at various ages.

Results of Reading Achievement Tests*

| | Age at Testing | | | |
Test	13	14	15	19
Stanford Achievement Test				
Paragraph meaning	2.4	3.9	3.5	3.5
Word meaning	3.0	2.0	3.5	4.0
Spelling	3.0	3.5	3.5	3.5
Gray Oral Paragraphs	1.6	2.9	3.5	4.0
Gates-MacGinitie Reading Tests	-	3.7	3.5	4.0

*Results are given in grade levels. At 6 years of age the patient's IQ (Stanford-Binet) was 105; at 13 years it was (WISC): full scale 88; verbal 95; nonverbal 83.

(From "Cytoarchitesctonic Abnormalities in Developmental Dyxlexia: A Case Study," by Albert M. Galaburda and Thomas L. Kemper, *Annals of Neurology*, 6, August 1979, p. 95. Used with permission.)

Note how very little progress was made in *six* years, with scarcely any between the ages of fifteen and nineteen. One wonders what kind of help he received, whether he was a visual or auditory dyslexic, or if the diagnostician knew the difference. Note that the diagnosis of dyslexia was made at an early age. Obviously his special tutoring did not help very much. When he was sixteen years old he developed nocturnal seizures, but these were easily controlled with phenytoin. No other member of his family had seizures. At age sixteen he had repeated neurological examinations, but no abnormalities were noted. And except for one sleep study indicating borderline slowing over the right hemisphere, routine electroencephalograms were normal. An isotope brain scan was also normal.

His arithmetic performance was thought to be better than his reading and spelling, but he scored at the fourth-grade level on an arithmetic assessment when he was eighteen years old. At this time it was noted that he had some mild problems with left-right orientation and finger recognition.

Dr. Galaburda and Dr. Kemper examined the young man's brain and found no gross abnormalities and no abnormalities in myelination, size of ventricles, nor thickness of the corpus callosum. The abnormalities that were found were all confined to the left cerebral hemisphere. Here, within the language areas, the doctors found a disordered cortex (the layer of gray matter covering most of the surface of the brain) with frequently fused layers, scrambled and whirled, and with numerous abnormally large cells scattered "throughout the thickness of the cortical ribbon, often extending into the subcortical white matter for a short distance." This abnormal neuronal architecture was found mainly in the areas of the brain which are concerned with the auditory region and language.[23]

In addition to the above, Galaburda and Kemper found that the planum temporale (temples) on both sides were symmetrical. (Usually the left is larger.) But the doctors pointed out that this finding likely did not represent an abnormality since such symmetry in the extent of the planum can occur in as many as 24 percent of normal persons.

Though the left cerebral hemisphere was consistently wider than the right hemisphere, the implications were not clear to the researchers. As the doctors pointed out:

> It is not possible to tell from a single case whether or not the an-atomical findings have any causative relationship to the clinical findings—much less whether the malformation is responsible for the seizure disorder, the learning disability, both, or neither.[24]

Cerebellar-Vestibular (C-V) Dysfunction

The theory that cerebellar-vestibular dysfunction is a cause of dyslexia is being treated separately and placed last in this chapter for a reason. I have mixed feelings about even presenting this notion, which has received quite a bit of press and television publicity, but which has been repudiated by neu-rologists, psychiatrists, educators, and organizations dealing with dyslexia. But in true education one must be aware of the thinking of others, must consider the issues and the facts, and must draw conclusions based upon knowledge and experience.

Harold N. Levinson, a psychiatrist, has written two books[25] setting forth his hypothesis. The first is rather technical, somewhat lengthy, and requires persistence to get through. The second book presents his information in a more readable manner for the general public.

First, some background information is needed to understand Levinson's theory about the cause of dyslexia. The cerebral cortex controls numerous muscles with the aid of the cerebellum, which has been called our biological computer. There are different kinds of activities which are performed by the cerebellum, but this one example will relate to Levinson's theory: try holding your index finger in a vertical position approximately six inches in front of your face. Then begin moving your hand from side to side as quickly as you can. What happened? Your finger became just a blur. Now try it from the op-posite approach: Hold your hand (and finger) very steadily while moving your head from side to side as fast as you can. Now what happened? There was much less blurring. The reason for this is that the *vestibul occular reflex* (VOR) largely prevented the blurring. The VOR extends from the *vestibular center* in the inner ear and served to keep your eyes on the fixed target of your finger as you moved your head from side to side.

Levinson holds that the root of dyslexia lies in this area; that is, an inner ear dysfunction that can be treated with varying degrees of dosage and combinations of medication, such as ritalin, dramamine, marezine, antivert, benedryl, as well as vitamins such as Vitamin B complex, B6, B12, Niacin, ginger root, and other chemicals and nutrients. He claims to have cured over ten thousand dyslexics in the past ten years with these drugs and nutrients.

Levinson reports that some of his "dyslexics" have been excellent readers and spellers in school, and he has "found" that all of his phobic patients have dyslexia. He devised an instrument called a 3-D Optical Scanner to measure eye-tracking defects, and this he uses as a diagnostic screening tool to detect "dyslexia." He asserts that 95 percent accuracy is obtained with this instrument, and that, with the medication, there is a remarkable improvement in schoolwork. He even claims that his medication has cured deafness and stuttering as well as dyslexia.

Some criticisms of Levinson's studies and work are as follows:

1. Dyslexia is a complex disability. Dyslexics have problems in reading, writing, spelling, listening, and speaking. They do *not* excel in schoolwork, as did some of Levinson's "dyslexics." So the first question must be whether his patients were truly dyslexic, or just persons with emotional problems, various phobias, psychosomatic disorders, hyperactivity, or other behavioral difficulties. One parent in Levinson's book was told that her daughter's "work, when she did it, was all above average."[26] *Dyslexics cannot do their work* at the expected grade levels—much less perform well above average.
2. No "double-blind" studies were done. A "double-blind" study is one in which some of the participants (the "control group") take "placebos" (such as sugar pills), while others are given the real medication under study. These studies are called double-blind because neither the participants nor the examiners know which is the phony pill and which is the real pill, though of course the directors of the research do.
3. Neurologists have criticized Levinson's neurological examinations, which identified cerebellar dysfunction, and have disputed that these can identify vestibular dysfunction.
4. The children who participated in the "Queens Study" blurring-speed experiment were kindergarten students. The question of visual and other developmental immaturity and the possible effect upon such young children must be raised, with the consequence of invalid results as far as dyslexia is concerned.

5. The children who participated in the "Staten Island Study" were students in nursery school, kindergarten, first and second grades. The same question regarding visual and other developmental immaturity must be asked.

6. Levinson later admitted that the results of the blurring speed studies were confounded by "unwittingly" comparing premedication with postmedication subjects.

Full Circle

We do not yet know all the causes of dyslexia. That it exists, we do know. Brain injury and certain illness can cause acquired dyslexia. Heredity plays a role in some cases of dyslexia, but how this occurs in some families is not known at the present time. In other words, the specific linkage has not been established. And, more boys than girls have dyslexia.

We are not going to make much progress in discovering the cause(s) of dyslexia until our diagnoses become more accurate, and experiments and other research tighten up. In a sense, progress in dyslexia knowledge may have been impeded by the "research, publish, or perish" dicta at our large universities. Too much hasty, sloppy, questionable research has been turned out. Longitudinal studies take *time*; any well-designed and well-researched study takes time and conscientious, intelligent, objective evaluation of the findings.

Somehow, this message must be gotten across to those who need to hear it if we are ever going to reach the end of the road. So far, the dyslexia route has been circular, tortuous, and frustrating.

Notes for Chapter 9

1. Knud Hermann, *Reading Disability, A Medical Study of Word-Blindness and Related Handicaps* (Springfield, Illinois: Charles C. Thomas, 1959), pp. 86–87.

2. Zerbin-Rubin, "Congenital Word Blindness," *Bulletin of the Orton Society* 17, (1967), p. 50.

3. Bertil Hallgren, *Specific Dyslexia ("Congenital Word-Blindness"): A Clinical and Genetic Study* (Copenhagen: Ejnar Munksgaard, 1950; trans. from the Swedish by Erica Odelberg, Stockholm: Esselte aktiebolag, 1950), p. 272.

4. Ibid., pp. 194–195.

5. Donald G. Doehring, *Patterns of Impairment in Specific Reading Disability, A Neuropsychological Investigation* (Bloomington: Indiana University Press, 1968), p. 83.

6. Edith Klasen, *The Syndrome of Specific Dyslexia* (Baltimore: University Park Press, 1972), p. 78.

7. Sandhya Naidoo, *Specific Dyslexia* (New York: John Wiley & Sons, 1972), pp. 96–97, III.

0. Joan M Finucci, John T. Guthrie, Anne L. Childs, Helen Abbey, and Barton Childs, "The Genetics of Specific Reading Disability," *Annals of Human Genetics* 40 (London, 1976), p. 17.

9. David Elkind, John Horn, and Gerrie Schneider, "Modified Word Recognition, Reading Achievement, and Perceptual De-centration," *Journal of Genetic Psychology* 107 (December 1965), p. 248.

10. Richard M. Restak, *The Brain* (New York: Bantam, 1984), p. 173.

11. Samuel T. Orton, " 'Word-blindness' in School Children," *Archives of Neurology and Psychiatry* 14, No. 5 (November 1925), pp. 607–609.

12. G. Keith Connors, "Critical Review of Electroencephalographic and Neurophysiological Studies in Dyslexia," Arthur L. Benton and David Pearl, eds. *Dyslexia, an Appraisal of Current Knowledge* (New York: Oxford University, 1978), p. 260.

13. T. T. S. Ingram, A. W. Mason, and J. Blackburn, "A Retrospective Study of 82 Children With Reading Disability," *Developmental Medicine and Child Neurology* 12 (1970), p. 280.

14. Connors' (1978) critique of EEG studies, op. cit., pp. 259–260:
   (a) Most studies employ nonblind readings of unknown reliability.
   (b) Studies vary in the definition of the dyslexic group.
   (c) Studies frequently do not rule out associated conditions such as behavior or neurological abnormalities.
   (d) Matching of experimental and control samples is usually poor, and where it is good there is no EEG-reading association.
   (e) More recent and well-controlled studies show significantly less abnormality than is reported for earlier studies.
   (f) The range of degree-of-abnormality reported is too large to inspire confidence in the reliability of the findings.
   (g) No consistent findings have appeared with respect to either the locus or type of abnormality associated with dyslexia.
   (h) In the cases where follow-up evaluations of EEG-studied dyslexics were performed, the EEG contributed nothing to prediction of outcome.
   (i) There are several instances where the greater degree of abnormality of the EEG is associated with the milder conditions of the reading disorder.
   (j) There are several instances where the greater degree of abnormality among the dyslexics is less than that found in other studies among controls.

15. Restak, op.cit., pp. 351–352.

16. Ibid., p. 352.

17. Ibid., p. 248.

18. Ibid., p. 250.

19. Ibid., pp. 250–251.

20. Ibid., pp. 250, 252, 257–260.

21. Bryon P. Rourke, Dirk J. Bakker, John L. Fisk, and John D. Strang, *Child Neuropsychology, An Introduction to Theory, Research and Clinical Practice* (New York: Guilford Press, 1983), pp. 104–105.

22. Albert M. Galaburda and Thomas L. Kemper, "Cytoarchitectonic Abnormalities in Developmental Dyslexia: A Case Study," *Annals of Neurology* Vol. 6 (August 1979), pp. 94–100.
23. Galaburda and Kemper, op.cit., p. 96.
24. Ibid., p. 99.
25. Harold N. Levinson, *A Solution to the Riddle Dyslexia* (New York: Springer-Verlag, 1980); *Smart But Feeling Dumb* (New York: Warner Books, 1984).
26. Levinson, (1984), op.cit., p. 58.

PART FOUR: DYSLEXIA IN ADOLESCENCE AND MATURITY

'Tis education forms the common mind:
Just as the twig is bent the tree's inclined.
—*Alexander Pope*

CHAPTER
10

DYSLEXIA IN THE MIDDLE SCHOOL AND HIGH SCHOOL

True, children are educable in varying
degrees, but the variation in degree must be
of the same kind and quality of education.
If "the best education for the best is the
best education for all," the failure to carry
out that principle is the failure on the part
of society—a failure of parents, of
teachers, of administrators—not a failure
on the part of the children.

—*Mortimer J. Adler*

If the dyslexia is not detected in the elementary school, remediation for the
dyslexic student tends to take longer and may be more difficult to achieve
because of his age. There are several reasons for this. The student's self-
esteem has been damaged over years of being unable to keep up with his fellow students in school or to satisfy the performance expectations of his teachers and his parents. Feelings of frustration and anxiety have built up inside him
as a result of continuing failure and low grades. His motivation and drive to
take on certain tasks is deadened. "What's the use?" he thinks. Since his difficulties have not been overcome or even ameliorated, he continues to

reinforce his incorrect responses to the point where they become internalized and automatic.

The older dyslexic often develops the pretense of not caring about the quality of his schoolwork or his grades. He may try to act superior, belittling or "putting down" those to whom he may feel inferior. He is thin-skinned, with a prickly personality, and is subject to irritability and verbal (and sometimes physical) explosions. He may burst out with a nasty retort and withdraw to his desk at school or to his room at home. By now he may have been diagnosed as "emotionally disturbed," and the underlying dyslexia may have become eclipsed by its own creation.

Often the middle school or high school dyslexic becomes a "loner." By evading social interchange he naively believes that he can prevent the other students from finding out that he cannot read the textbooks, cannot perform as he thinks they do. Each year in school the gap increases between his chronological age and his academic achievement—unless he gets the help he needs—and his social withdrawal is likely to become more pronounced.

The lecture method of instruction is common in middle and high school classes. And of course the dyslexic student has difficulty listening to a lecture, following the sequence of what the teacher is saying, remembering what he has heard. He has trouble recording the notes of the lecture because of his problems with immediate recall, sequencing, spelling, and writing. His lecture notes are likely to be scanty, disorganized, in bits and pieces, and are almost impossible to study for a review. The faster the teacher talks (or reads), the more confused the dyslexic's notes become.

Some middle and high school teachers fill the chalkboards with notes prior to class and expect the students to spend a large part of the period copying the notes for future study. Often diagrams or charts must also be copied. All of this is very difficult for the visual dyslexic. So too is copying notes or diagrams from the overhead projector which teachers in the upper grades frequently use, for the student has to look up repeatedly to see the material, then look down at his paper to reproduce it. His visual memory and integration problems interfere with the smooth transference of letters, words, and punctuation. He must work slowly. Often he does not complete the copying, usually to the dismay of his teacher. A teacher may also find it hard to understand the errors in copying, since "it is all right there in front of you!" or the messiness, which is a tendency of both visual and auditory dyslexics.

School essays, book reports, science or social studies reports, and other such projects present special problems to the older dyslexic. But by this age, he has developed certain "survival techniques" (sometimes called "avoidance techniques") as a result of receiving papers covered with red ink corrections— sometimes with sarcastic remarks about his numerous errors and sloppiness in spelling and handwriting—and the inevitable low grades. (He writes as little as possible, using only those words that he thinks he knows how to spell, or he plagiarizes, although he makes some errors in copying.)

Scores on tests and examinations may be low because of his reading and writing problems in class. They may also be low, not because he does not know the answers, but because he is unable to read the significant words in the questions or because his short-term memory and sequencing problems distort his perception of what is being asked. It is only the few and fortunate dyslexic students who are placed with an understanding teacher (who has a caring, courageous, and supportive principal), who is allowed to read and clarify test questions for them, or who will take the time to tape the questions of a test. When this is done the dyslexic student benefits by looking at the words of the directions as he hears them being spoken.

The dyslexic student needs additional time in which to write his answers because of his mental processing problems and his slow handwriting rate. If he can speak the answers to the questions softly into a tape recorder for the teacher to check later, the result will be a more realistic assessment of the student's progress.

The dyslexic student is, obviously, likely to have trouble with foreign languages in high school. The elimination of foreign language requirements by many colleges and universities may have distressed educators, foreign service personnel, and others, but it has been a great help to the dyslexic who seeks higher education. For the auditory dyslexic, a foreign language may present an impossible task. For the visual dyslexic, writing the language is the hurdle that must be overcome, not speaking it. Some visual dyslexics have learned to speak a foreign language by ear; that is, by living in a foreign country or by participating in a conversation class that requires no writing.

The older visual dyslexic student finds geometry trying, with the need to reproduce various geometric designs, compare figures, take measurements, and write logical proofs. Depending upon the degree of severity and the type of dyslexia, band, chorus, and music appreciation classes may be difficult because of the need to read musical notations, to keep in step during precision drills, and simply to keep in time. Visual dyslexic students have trouble with algebra mainly because of transposition and sequencing problems.

Secondary school teachers should take a page from the elementary teacher's book of methods. Rather than predominantly using the lecture method in the classroom, the "unit" method of teaching would be most successful with the dyslexic student. This technique can be used for *any* subject. Here the students are not sitting passively at their desks taking or copying notes but are *actively* involved in the instruction through various shared activities, planning, demonstrating, and so on. Books containing the basic concepts but written at lower reading levels are used. Even more telling, rather than having a single textbook at one level for all students in a class (no matter the level of their reading), there is a variety of books on the curriculum topics, and at differing reading levels.

Some teacher-training institutions require a knowledge of unit teaching by their graduates, but too often they leave this knowledge at the college, either because they are employed by a school system that mandates a single textbook in a class or does not provide the funds for a variety of books at differing levels, or because the teachers give in to the simpler and less time-consuming use of one textbook and let it dictate what is to be taught and how it is to be taught. It is unfortunate when the teacher becomes the tool and the textbook the master. It is the student who suffers.

By law, students are required to remain in school until a certain age. As a result of "social promotion" (because of age) students are moved to the next grade, sometimes after repeating a year or more in elementary school. But all children in a particular grade, say the tenth grade, are not reading at the tenth grade level. In a typical tenth-grade class, the range of reading levels is likely to cover a span of seven grades or more. Yet it is common practice for schools to adopt a single textbook for each subject for each grade level. All students are expected to read the same textbook both in and out of class, whether or not the reading level makes for ease of reading and understanding. No wonder so many middle and high school teachers feel frustrated when they haven't the least idea what to do with the students who cannot read the required textbook.

According to the latest *NASDTEC MANUAL* (Manual on Certification and Preparation of Educational Personnel in the United States), a course, such as the teaching of reading or applying reading to a high school subject, is neither specified nor required of any secondary teacher seeking certification in twelve of our fifty states. Four states include reading only as one of a group of courses that *may* be taken, which means that some other course may be elected in its place. Three states require a reading course for English teachers only. One state requires this of only English and social studies teachers. One requires the course for all teachers except those in art, home economics, industrial arts, music, or physical education. Another merely states that whether a reading course is taken depends on "the endorsement obtained and renewal period." [1] Only twenty-eight states require the teaching of reading or reading in the content areas for all secondary school certification. Here is another reason our dyslexic students have been falling by the wayside. In addition to notetaking problems during lectures, they have problems with the textbooks and the required reading in their classes.

During the upper level school years, nearly 90 percent of a student's studies will depend upon his reading achievement.[2] As a result, the dyslexic public high school student often ends up in vocational shop classes. Early diagnosis of the problem with the necessary treatment to alleviate the disability would help many capable and highly motivated dyslexics move toward a higher education.

What About College for the Dyslexic?

Of course it is possible for a dyslexic to attend college, although his preferred college may not be the best for him. The degree of his success in college will depend to a considerable extent upon the severity of his dyslexic condition. It will also depend upon his intelligence, interest, motivation, drive, self-discipline, persistence, health, and energy level.

Special tutoring will probably be necessary, and this will add to the cost of college. Often this can be provided by another college student who has done especially well in a particular course in which the dyslexic needs help. A typewriter for term papers and special reports is essential. Better yet, hire a typist for this job (more cost to the dyslexic student). Help in proofreading anything handwritten is essential, but both the help and the reason for it should be made known to the professor.

Learning to use a word processor could be helpful for the dyslexic student in writing papers, particularly if it included the spelling correction programs, although these do not catch all the misspellings. Proofreading would still be necessary. For example, if one were to write "he went into the house" as "he went in to the house," the spelling program would not pick up the word because *into, in* and *to* are all correctly spelled. In other words, certain "usage" errors are not picked up. If the student were to use certain words that are not in the program, they too may not be picked up for correction.

Little research has been done with longitudinal and follow-up studies of dyslexics—testing students in elementary school and then following up and retesting them as adults to determine their academic progress, educational attainments, and occupational status. We also need ongoing (not retroactive) information about: the kinds of remedial help being given; the frequency of remediation instruction and whether it is on a one-to-one or group basis (and size of group); whether the students remain in regular classrooms and receive special remedial help or spend all day in special classes; the yearly progress of each student. Ongoing, progressive records of such information are highly preferable to retroactive information with its many gaps.

The information obtained from the few follow-up studies that have been done is contradictory. It leaves one in doubt about what really can be expected of the dyslexic. Of course, the severity of the condition, the time of the diagnosis, the quality and amount of remedial help, the intelligence of the dyslexic, and various personality factors previously mentioned, combine to affect the progress of a dyslexic student and his future life. Then, too, one must consider the accuracy of the diagnoses when considering the progress of students who have fallen behind for one reason or another.

Forty young men who had been diagnosed as being dyslexic at the Hawthorn Center, a mental health facility in Michigan for children and adolescents, were retested to determine their academic progress over approximately ten years after they were first diagnosed.[3] They continued to have serious diffi-culty, and many of the types of errors noted earlier persisted. The highest read ing level score of these men was 8.4 (eighth grade, fourth month). The highest spelling level score was 6.6 (sixth grade, sixth month). These reading and spelling levels are not likely to gain one admission to college, much less allow one to succeed in college after getting there.

Several aspects should be noted about this study. The Wechsler Intelli-gence Scale for Children (WISC) was administered at the time of diagnosis. The Verbal IQs varied from 66 to 103, with Full Scale IQs varying from 80 to 112. No follow-up Wechsler Adult Intelligence Scale (WAIS) was given. The re-searcher does not indicate the number of students at each level of intelligence, and if the range of IQs was skewed to the left—more scores falling at the lower end of the scale—one cannot expect the same amount and rate of prog-ress for those of lower intelligence as for those of higher intelligence. Some of the symptoms of low intelligence are similar to those of dyslexia (poor se-quencing, some reversals, problems with abstract concepts, immature draw-ings, poor auditory discrimination, and so on). Were some of the participants in this study simply slow learners, or slow learning dyslexics?

The quantity and quality of remedial help is not known. Remedial help was defined as assistance by specially trained persons in a group of ten or fewer outside the classroom two or three times a week. But the *total* amount of remediation given each dyslexic *varied tremendously*, ranging from only one to five semesters for nine students to sixteen to twenty-four semesters for six students. (The researcher "concluded" that there was no relationship be-tween the amount of reading assistance and the adult reading levels!)

In contrast to the above study, published in 1978, in a prior follow-up study, published in 1968, of twenty dyslexic boys[4] (eight "moderately" dyslexic and twelve "severely" dyslexic), most of them were found to have progressed steadily through secondary school. Three severe and two moderate dyslexics repeated grades, but all graduated from high school. All but two went on to graduate from college. Four completed a year of graduate study, one earned a law degree, one a graduate degree in divinity, and three were doctoral can-didates. Five had their doctoral degrees.

What happened to these dyslexic boys? Why had they not fallen by the wayside? There may be several reasons. Their dyslexia was diagnosed at a fairly early age and special help was given. The researcher, Rawson, states that one of this particular school's most valuable contributions was "to the self-concepts of the boys, a persistent faith in their intelligence and capacity to achieve, trans-mitted to the boys directly and indirectly."[5] The home environment must have had a great deal of influence. The families were "professionally oriented, highly educated, intelligent, 'intellectual,' upper-middle-class, financially solvent but not wealthy, educationally nonconventional, and individualistic." [6] The range of IQs was from average to superior—no slow learners.

One must add that this is a rather old study, and the boys were diagnosed as being "dyslexic" while still in elementary school. Much less was known about diagnosing dyslexia at that time, and it is possible that some of these boys were not dyslexic at all. No mention was made about the types of dyslexia.

The students in the above study began receiving help to alleviate their difficulties at a fairly early age. But the middle school or high school dyslexic who was not diagnosed at an earlier age can take heart from Vice President Nelson A. Rockefeller who, a dyslexic himself, had an interesting story to tell about his travels through the Land of Dyslexia Frustration and about his decision in the ninth grade to tackle his problem. He wrote the following article in connection with a television special called "The Puzzle Children." Older students will be able to identify with some of his experiences:

Don't Accept Anyone's Verdict That You Are Lazy, Stupid or Retarded

By Vice President Nelson A. Rockefeller

Those watching the Public Broadcasting Service program on "The Puzzle Children" will include a very interested vice president of the United States.

For I was one of the "puzzle children" myself—a dyslexic, or "reverse reader"—and I still have a hard time reading today.

But after coping with this problem for more than 60 years, I have a message of encouragement for children with learning disabilities—and their parents.

Based on my own experience, my message to dyslexic children is this:

— Don't accept anyone's verdict that you are lazy, stupid or retarded. You may very well be smarter than most other children your age . . .

— You can learn to cope with your problem and turn your so-called disability into a positive advantage.

Dyslexia forced me to develop powers of concentration that have been invaluable throughout my career in business, philanthropy and public life.

And I've done an enormous amount of reading and public speaking, especially in political campaigns for governor of New York and president of the United States.

No one had ever heard of dyslexia when I discovered as a

boy, along about the third grade, that reading was such a difficult chore that I was in the bottom one-third of my class.

None of the educational, medical and psychological help available today for dyslexics was available in those days.

We had no special teachers or tutors, no special classes or courses, no special methods of teaching—because nobody understood our problem.

Along with an estimated three million other children, I just struggled to understand words that seemed to garble before my eyes, numbers that came out backwards, sentences that were hard to grasp.

And so I accepted the verdict . . . that I wasn't as bright as most of the rest of my class at the Lincoln School in New York City. Fortunately for me, the school (though it never taught me to spell!) was an experimental, progressive institution with the flexibility to let you develop your own interests and follow them.

More to the point, I had a wise and understanding counselor in Dr. Otis W. Caldwell, the headmaster.

"Don't worry," he said, "just because you're in the lower third of the class. You've got the intelligence. If you just work harder and concentrate more, you can make it."

So I learned, through self-discipline, to concentrate, which in my opinion is essential for a dyslexic.

While I could speak better French than the teacher, because I'd learned it as a child, I couldn't conjugate the verbs. I did flunk Spanish—but now can speak it fluently because I learned it by ear, later, at the Berlitz School.

My best subject was mathematics; I understood concepts well beyond my grade level. But it took only one reversed number in a column of figures to cause havoc.

When I came close to flunking out in the ninth grade—because I didn't work very hard that year—I decided that I had better follow Dr. Caldwell's advice if I wanted to go to college.

I even told my high-school girl friend that we would have to stop dating so I could spend the time studying in order to get into Dartmouth.

And I made it by the skin of my teeth.

I made it simply by working harder and longer than the rest—eventually learning to concentrate sufficiently to compensate for my dyslexia in reading.

I adopted a regimen of getting up at 5 A.M. to study, and studying without fail. And thanks to my concentration and the very competitive nature I was born with, I found my academic performance gradually improving . . .

I owe a great debt to my professors and to President Erneste M. Hopkins. I had met Dr. Hopkins earlier and was so impressed that I had made Dartmouth my goal. Most of all, however, I think I owe my academic improvement to my roommate, Johnny French.

Johnny and I were the exact opposites. He was reticent, and had the highest IQ in the class. To me, he was that maddening type who got straight A's with only occasional reference to books or classes. He was absolutely disgusted by my study habits—anybody who got up at 5 in the morning to hit the books was, well, peculiar.

Inevitably, Johnny made Phi Beta Kappa in our junior year, but my competitive instincts kept me going. We were both elected to senior fellowships and I made Phi Beta Kappa in my senior year . . .

Looking back over the years, I remember vividly the pain and mortification I felt as a boy of 8, when I was assigned to read a short passage of Scripture at a community vesper service during summer vacation in Maine—and did a thoroughly miserable job of it.

I know what a dyslexic child goes through—the frustration of not being able to do what other children do easily, the humiliation of being thought not too bright when such is not the case at all.

My personal discoveries as to what is required to cope with dyslexia could be summarized in these admonitions to the individual dyslexic:

Accept the fact that you have a problem—don't just try to hide it.

Refuse to feel sorry for yourself.

Realize that you don't have an excuse—you have a challenge.

Face the challenge.

Work harder and learn mental discipline—the capacity for total concentration—and

Never quit.

If it helps a dyslexic child to know I went through the same thing . . .

But can conduct press conferences today in three languages . . .

And can read a speech on television . . .

(Though I may have to rehearse it six times . . .

(With my script in large type . . .

(And my sentences broken into segments like these . . .

(And long words broken into syllables) . . .

And I have learned to read and communicate well enough to be elected Governor of New York four times . . .

And to win Congressional confirmation as Vice President of the United States . . .

Then I hope the telling of my story as a dyslexic could be an inspiration to the "puzzle children"—for that's what I really care about.[7]

Rockefeller had "true grit" and self-discipline, plus high intelligence and a goal very important to him. He did not have auditory dyslexia and was able to do much learning by ear, as evidenced by his learning to speak Spanish at the Berlitz School and to speak French as a child. *Writing* the language was another story because of his visual dyslexia, which also contributed to his problems in math and reading.

In Rockefeller's school days, very little, if anything, was known about dyslexia by most of those in education. Today, there is no excuse for anyone connected with the education of children to be ignorant of this disability. School priorities may need to be reorganized so that dyslexics will be detected and receive the help they need. This means that trained reading specialists must be at the elementary, middle, and high school levels to detect dyslexics and to work with them. New lights or an enlarged stadium or new band uniforms may need to take a lower priority if necessary to enable the business of educating all the children in our schools to proceed in our democratic society.

The College Board: Services for Dyslexic Students

Since 1939, the College Board has made available special editions of its tests for handicapped students. These include students with dyslexia. Special editions of the Scholastic Achievement Test (SAT) and the Test of Standard Written English (TSWE) may be administered with extended time to dyslexic students. They may also work with cassettes and may use a typewriter or an abacus, but not a calculator.

The need for a special test must be documented by an individual educational plan that states the nature and effect of the handicap as well as the modified testing arrangements required. In the absence of such documentation and plan, statements signed by qualified personnel must be provided describing the handicap and the need for a special testing arrangement.

The high school counselor should order the tests, answer sheets, and practice materials, and should request the cassettes from Educational Testing Service (ETS) in Princeton, New Jersey.[8]

Notes for Chapter 10

1. *The NASDTEC Manual* (Manual on Certification and Preparation of Educational Personnel in the United States), National Association of State Directors of Teacher Education and Certification, Robert A. Roth and Richard Mastain, eds. (1984), pp. G-6 through G-8.
2. Herman K. Goldberg, Gilbert B. Schiffman, and Michael Bender, *Dyslexia, Interdisciplinary Approaches to Reading Disabilities* (New York: Grune and Stratton, 1983), p. 6.
3. John G. Frauenheim, "Academic Achievement Characteristics of Adult Males Who Were Diagnosed as Dyslexic in Childhood," *Journal of Learning Disabilities* 2 (October 1978), pp. 21–28.
4. Margaret B. Rawson, *Developmental Language Disability: Adult Accomplishments of Dyslexic Boys* (Baltimore: Johns Hopkins, 1968), pp. 74, 76.
5. Ibid., p. 110.
6. Ibid., p. 109.
7. Nelson Rockefeller, "Don't Accept Anyone's Verdict That You Are Lazy, Stupid or Retarded," *TV Guide* (October 16, 1978), pp. 12–14. Reprinted with permission from TV GUIDE® Magazine. Copyright © 1976 by Triangle Publications, Inc., Radnor, Pennsylvania.
8. "Information for Students with Special Needs," Admissions Testing Program, College Entrance Examination Board, Princeton, New Jersey (1984), pp. 1–4.

CHAPTER
11

THE ADULT DYSLEXIC IN OUR SOCIETY

There are golden ages yet to be made and
times of trouble to be survived. The book is
a shield, a tool and a power-pack. It is an
instrument for intellectual and emotional
navigation. It is men's own sovereign remedy
against the ills and confusions of a changing
universe. The more competent readers a
society has, the greater will be its capacity
for doing good itself. Wakeful happiness
should be the best condition of men.
—*Frank G. Jennings*

There is no way of determining the number of adult dyslexics in our society. Many are part of that larger number of functionally illiterate adults
who are unable to perform productively as citizens, family members,
consumers, or workers. The National Commission on Literacy has reported
that 30 million adult Americans cannot read a want ad or a newspaper. One of
five high school seniors cannot perform basic reading tasks upon graduation.[1]
The United States Census Bureau defines as illiterate a person who is at least
fourteen years old but who has not finished the fifth grade. But this standard
no longer holds true, for the reading levels of American newspapers and wire
services range from the eleventh grade to the level of college freshmen[2]—not

the fourth or fifth grade level, as some previously thought.

A sixth grade reading level is needed to understand a driver's license manual. An eighth grade reading level is necessary to follow the directions for cooking a TV dinner and to read the federal income tax form. A tenth grade reading level is needed to understand the directions on an aspirin bottle, and a twelfth grade reading level to read and understand an insurance policy.[3]

In answer to a class action suit brought by Legal Services for the Elderly against Medicare in the federal court in New York, a letter sent by Medicare to claimants was found to have a readability level that ranged from the twelfth to the sixteenth grade (college senior). The court found that 48 percent of the residents of New York age sixty-five and older have an eighth grade education or less.[4]

When the adult dyslexic enrolls his children in school and is asked their dates of birth he may not be able to recall them. This is likely to shock the school recorder. Often I have heard the remark, "Would you believe that man doesn't even know when his children were born? Doesn't he *care* about his family?" She would be even more surprised to know that the same person may not remember the date of his marriage, when he had that car accident, or in what order he was supposed to stop by the classroom, the secretary's office, and the principal's office. And none has a thing to do with caring for his family.

The adult dyslexic has trouble using the telephone directory, dictionaries, encyclopedias, and other indices, and filing papers because of his problems with alphabetical order and spelling. For this he needs a competent secretary.

The adult visual dyslexic should keep a small pocket notebook in which he can make notes or keep lists to use as a check on what he needs to do and when he is supposed to do them. For some, a digital watch may be easier to read than the ordinary type that has two (sometimes three) hands and twelve numbers, and because of his sequencing difficulties. Care must be taken, though, when reading the numbers that these are not transposed and thus read out of order—12:15 read as 12:51—and of course reversals can still occur—9:26 becomes 6:29 or 9:56 becomes 6:59. Some modern watches have only dots or lines to indicate where the numerals should be. These, too, may present problems for the visual dyslexic because he must draw on memory and visual imagery to place the appropriate numerals and count the minutes (in sequence). A wristwatch with an alarm will help remind the dyslexic of appointments and time schedules. Here again, care must be taken when setting the alarm that the correct numerals are used. Double-checking the setting should be habitual.

A dyslexic artillery observer might confuse the numbers in his map coordinates and call down fire on his own forces!

Reading road maps or traveling by train or bus or the subways can be troublesome. The dyslexic may need to record the stops in his notebook before his destination and refer to them as he travels. He may wish to ask the conductor or bus driver to announce his stop. He should *never* be hesitant to ask someone for help if in doubt.

The visual dyslexic must use a calculator with caution and much double-checking because visual memory, transposition and other reversal errors, and sequencing problems may result in tabulating inaccurate information. Still, it will probably be more accurate than trying to figure without a calculator. Referring to and copying from sets of mathematical tables can result in serious mistakes for the same reasons.

Obviously, reversals and sequencing errors with numerals can lead to mistakes in the preparation of income tax returns. I would advise the dyslexic to have someone check his figures.

When participating in parades, whether military or otherwise, the adult dyslexic may confuse right with left and have difficulty keeping in step. Piloting an airplane could be very dangerous. In one example of this, there was a case where certain pilots seemed to be involved in a large number of accidents or incidents in the air force. A psychologist, Gerhardt, was asked to investigate the matter. He discovered that many of the pilots often confused right and left directions (and also were poor readers and spellers),[5] with disastrous consequences when they had to make quick decisions concerning a right or left action.

Learning a special code, such as the Morse Code, is a difficult task for both the visual and auditory dyslexic. Accurate sequencing of coded symbols is necessary, and dots and dashes must be in correct order.

When writing an Incident Report, policemen must relate the occurrence of events in accurate order. Indeed, included in the multiple-choice examination given to applicants by the New York City Police Department are tests requiring the applicants to place disconnected sentences in "logical order."[6]

Reading the subtitles used with foreign movies is frustrating to the dyslexic because the lines are exposed for too short a time for him to be able to process the information.

Can Adult Dyslexics Be Helped?

Motivation, drive, a strong need to learn, and a willingness to work hard and long will speed the adult's remediation. He usually feels that time is passing him by, giving a sense of urgency to his attitude.

A young man in his early thirties, "S", called and asked for help. He was a salesman—energetic, likeable, convincing, and doing well at his job. Why did he need help? He had been offered a promotion with the firm for whom he worked, but he knew he would be unable to read and write the necessary reports. Up to that time his wife had been writing out all his orders for him from notes he made on a pad.

But his wife could hardly follow him into the office and be his help-mate there as she had been at home. He wanted to accept the offer very much because it would mean less traveling, which he did not enjoy. He said that he was under constant strain to get where he was going—not just to the particular town or city, but even to the business office on which he was supposed to call. This was especially difficult if the place were strange to him.

The young man came in for the necessary series of diagnostic tests. Findings indicated a moderate degree of visual dyslexia. A conference was set up with "S" and his wife to discuss several possibilities of action. I was impressed with his wife's genuine desire to help her husband in any way she could. She said that helping him kept her busy and made her feel important in his life. She obviously admired her husband for what he was trying to do. Their relationship was one of warmth and mutual trust. Both had a sense of humor and could laugh at some of their experiences in life.

I was relieved to hear that in the new job "S" would have the services of a secretary although he had to share her with another employee. The secretary had been trained to use a dictating machine, and he was able to requisition one for his office. Having a secretary meant that he would have help with making telephone calls, typing, filing information folders and letters—and retrieving them from the files when needed. He could dictate letters, reports, memoranda, and the like. If he needed to bring home any papers or reports, his wife would help him.

We also set up a practical "crash" program of remediation, working first on urgent needs. "S" was a young man of high intelligence, healthy, energetic, disciplined, and certainly highly motivated. With these attributes working for him he could see some progress within a reasonably short time. This encouraged him to work even harder.

I am no longer working with "S," who was transferred to another city, but I do hear from him occasionally, and he and his wife are coping with the situation well. There remains a residual of difficulty—and there probably always will be—but this young man's success can serve as an inspiration for others who find themselves in similar situations.

The Center for Social Organization of Schools and certain members of the Department of Pediatrics at The Johns Hopkins University have done a study of adult dyslexics that gives encouraging results.[7] It was a large-scale, long-term follow-up of several hundred men who had attended the Gow School in South Wales, New York, graduating in the years 1940 through 1977.

Gow is a college preparatory school with grades seven through twelve. Students come from all over the United States to attend this boarding school for dyslexic boys. Most of the boys in the study had repeated a school grade before entering Gow. More than two-thirds attended Gow for at least two years, with several returning to their regular high schools at home. Average IQ of those in the study was 118 as measured by the Stanford-Binet Scale which was administered to the students while at Gow. Only 3.3 percent had an IQ score of 100 or below.[8]

About half of the Gow alumni have only a high school diploma. Of those with a college education, only a few have advanced degrees.[9] Over 80 percent of the Gow men have white collar jobs. Sixty percent of these are professionals or managers—but of the professionals, only a few are lawyers or physicians. Most are technicians or school teachers. Some of those in managerial or sales work are vice presidents, presidents, or chief executive officers. Many are owners of small businesses such as retail stores, construction work, and real estate.[10]

Attending Gow is not inexpensive. These men came from homes of sufficient means to allow them to attend this boarding school.

Can dyslexics be successful as adults? The answer is yes. But this yes must be qualified with the statement that there is no doubt that high intelligence and advantaged social backgrounds can weigh the scales in their favor, both as to the degree of success and the opportunity. Nevertheless, determination, discipline, and a willingness to work hard—true grit—are almost as important. The adult dyslexic can be helped and can succeed if he is willing to put in the time and effort. Again, the severity of the dyslexia, previous experiences in coping with the difficulty, the amount and quality of any remediation that may have been received—all will affect the level of accomplishment of the dyslexic adult.

Which Career to Choose?

It is just plain common sense to consider a vocation in which dyslexics can succeed. True, dyslexics may *possibly* become lawyers or even physicians, but these vocations pose special problems with the reading, writing, spelling, speaking, and listening involved in the academic preparation and the career itself. Not only the severity of the dyslexia, but the level of intelligence and the personality of the individual must be taken into account.

The dyslexic might give thought to sales work or certain technician jobs or managerial positions (if secretaries are available). I have some serious reservations about recommending the teaching profession to dyslexics. Teachers have a responsibility to serve as models for their students whenever speaking or reading to them and also in writing, whether on their papers, or on the chalkboard, or in notes sent home to their parents. Then too, they must listen and respond carefully to students. Their instruction must be presented in an organized manner with clarity and preciseness of thought. Ambiguity and disorganized lessons will not result in successful learning on the part of the students.

If a teacher should spell a word incorrectly on the chalkboard or on a student's paper, the child may be confused and learn the incorrect spelling of the word, especially if he is to copy the word on paper. Reversals of numerals in arithmetic will, of course, add to the general confusion.

Students in kindergarten and the primary grades must develop a left-to-right/top-to-bottom directional orientation, since this is how we read and write in our society. In physical education or in band-marching practice, miscalled directions concerning left or right could result in real chaos.

Students must learn the sequencing of ideas, events, and numbers, and apply this to all subjects. But how can they if their teacher is unable to do it accurately?

But here again, one must consider the severity of the dyslexia, the level of intelligence, and the personality of the individual.

The Adult Dyslexic and His Family

We cannot leave this section on the adult dyslexic without some specific comments about how this condition may affect the family. What about the emotional development of the children? Are there adjustments that must be made by the wife (or husband)? By the children?

These questions cannot be answered in a few words nor by a flat yes or no. Each case is different. The answers depend on many things: how serious the dyslexic condition is, whether it was diagnosed early, the extent of effective remediation, the emotional stability of the dyslexic and that of the spouse, the self-esteem of the family as a whole, how they perceive the dyslexia problem, and the mutual caring and respect and love that exists among the family members.

Earlier in this chapter I mentioned the willingness of the wife of "S" to help her husband with his job, and his endeavors to seek help and work at improving his condition. What will happen when the children begin arriving and the young wife has less time for her husband's work? Will he understand? Will he feel threatened and insecure? Will feelings of resentment build up in her because of the many demands upon her time? Will the children, as they enter school and learn to read and write, note their father's difficulties? Will they think less of him? Be embarrassed by his problem? Will the father try to hide his problems from them?

(In the case of this particular young family, I do believe that the young couple will cope well with the increased responsibility of children and the support needed by all.)

Little research has been done on the dyslexic's family as a whole to determine what happens in such families and how the members respond to each other as a result of having a dyslexic in the family. Psychologists Lenkowsky and Saposnek[11] have done a case history on a dyslexic male where the family almost fell apart. Mr. White was a thirty-five-year-old dyslexic, a high school graduate, who earned $16,000 a year as a respected trouble-shooter machinist for a major automotive industry. His innate intelligence helped him get through school where it seems he managed to talk his way out of situations that required reading. His teachers continued to pass him to the next higher grade, until he graduated from high school.

He developed a plan to set up a campground on municipal property, but since he was unable to draw or read blueprints accurately, he had to explain the project to the city officials while actually on the grounds. Here he would walk to the various spots and point where different structures should go and where the plumbing pipes would lie.

At work in the machine shop he had to devise a mnemonic (memory) ritual to locate objects on the job since he could not read the inventory lists.

No one knew of his inability to read other than his immediate family, his reading tutor, and a few psychotherapists whom he had seen. This secrecy required the complicity of the other members of his family, especially his wife, who had to take care of budget decisions, bank transactions, paying the bills, ordering meals in restaurants, and other tasks which require reading and writing.

As time passed, Mr. White saw himself increasingly in a role dependent and subordinate to his wife. He felt inadequate, unmasculine, and helpless. When frustrated, he frequently gave in to fits of rage during which he would break the furniture or become physically violent to his family, much to his wife's resentment. She also resented his insistent demands for praise for whatever he did. She began to treat him less like a husband and more like a child.

As so often happens when husbands and wives are at odds with one another, Mrs. White drew closer to their two daughters. The husband became more like a peer to the children, and he began to think of his wife as a strict, stern parent. He felt guilt-ridden and incompetent. The relationship deteriorated to the point where almost all their time together was spent in fighting. The older daughter, Susan, age fifteen, aware of the precarious balance of her parents' marriage, began to delve into drugs, made some token suicide attempts, and became promiscuous. She perceived that her actions united her parents in an attempt to help her.

Eventually Susan ended up in a state hospital, committed by her parents and diagnosed as having "sociopathic trait disturbance with mild schizophrenic tendencies." While Susan was away, the younger daughter started to assume Susan's mediator role with the parents. When Susan's stay in the hospital was prolonged, Mr. White lost control and threw his younger daughter and wife out of the house, threatened suicide with a gun to his head, and set flares around the house. He was hospitalized and diagnosed as a "paranoid schizophrenic with sociopathic tendencies." Upon his release, he lived alone for a while but then returned home.

When Susan was in turn finally released from the hospital, the family was referred for outpatient family therapy. The father was encouraged to seek help in learning to read, and family relationships were improved during the sessions as each began to understand what had happened to the family unit—and the reasons why.

This case history is rather extreme and probably atypical of most cases of dyslexia. For here the father, while a dyslexic, did not have the emotional stability essential for successful family relationships. In this case too, the father tried to hide his problem rather than bring it out in the open and get help, as did "S." In addition to having dyslexia, Mr. White was paranoid schizophrenic! No wonder his family had difficulties. Even had Mr. White not had dyslexia, I doubt that life would have been "normal" for the White family.

How can anyone unable to read manage to graduate from high school? I cannot answer this question. That it does happen, I know. How can a student go through twelve years of school and not have dyslexia diagnosed? This, too, I cannot answer. Again, I know it does happen.

Mr. White's dyslexia had not been diagnosed in school, and thus he received no remedial help to alleviate the condition. But then, neither had Nelson Rockefeller, who, in spite of his frustrations in school, retained a stable personality and faced up to his problems squarely while still in school, resolving to tackle the situation rather than designing ways to avoid certain requirements.

True grit can pay off for the dyslexic. Emotional stability is a must if he is to achieve lasting, caring relationships with others and achieve a rewarding place in society.

Notes for Chapter 11

1. *Written Word, An AAAA Project to Promote Communication in the Field of Functional Illiteracy* (Lincoln, Nebraska: AAAA Contact Center, May 1979).
2. John Micklos, "Reading Levels of Newspapers," *Reading '84* 1 (Newark, Delaware: International Reading Association, February 1984), p. 3.
3. "Ahead: A Nation of Illiterates?" *U.S. News and World Report* (May 17, 1982), pp. 53–55.
4. "Poor Writing Can Have Legal Consequences," *Reading Today* 2 (Newark, Delaware: International Reading Association, December 1984–January 1985), p. 7.
5. Michael Thomson, *Developmental Dyslexia* (Baltimore: Edward Arnold, 1984), p. 221.
6. "Readings . . . Finding New York's Finest," *Harper's* (February 1986), pp. 16-18. Apparently, the significance of testing for sequencing ability was lost upon those who quoted those items in this selection.

7. Linda S. Gottfredson, Joan M. Finucci, and Barton Childs "The Adult Occupational Success of Dyslexic Boys: A Large Scale, Long-Term Follow Up," Report No. 334 (Baltimore: Center for Social Organization of Schools, The Johns Hopkins University, March 1983), p. 8.
8. Ibid., p. 9.
9. Ibid., p. 57.
10. Ibid., p. 56.
11. Linda Klein Lenkowsky and Donald T. Saposnek, "Family Consequences of Parental Dyslexia," *Journal of Learning Disabilities* 11 (January 1978), pp. 60–64.

CHAPTER

12

SOME NOTABLE PEOPLE: DYSLEXIC OR NOT?

A man should never be ashamed to own he
has been in the wrong, which is but saying,
in other words, that he is wiser today than
he was yesterday.
                                        —*Alexander Pope*

Behold the turtle: he makes progress
only when he sticks his neck out.
                                        —*James B. Conant*

Nelson Rockefeller, former vice president of the United States, was a notable person who was able to overcome the handicap of dyslexia. His article, reproduced in the previous chapter, reflects the heartache of a boy who was having trouble in school but did not understand why. It also reflects the courage of a young student who decided that he was going to do something about his problem, the success he achieved, and how he continually had to cope with the problem.

Frequently, in books and articles on dyslexia, writers report a number of notable adults reputed to have had dyslexia. Repetition of these names has become almost a litany. These names are usually just listed in a series in books with rarely any explanation or evidence given why the person is considered to have been dyslexic. The few times any evidence is given it is scanty—often irrelevant or questionable. The problem here seems to be one of follow-the-leader and self-perpetuation. A writer mentions that it is possible that so-and-so *may* have had dyslexia. Another writer picks up the name and goes on to state that such-and-such *did* have dyslexia. And so it goes.

Yet in our desire to reassure and to give hope to the dyslexic himself and to the parents of dyslexic children, we must ever be on guard as professionals to avoid perpetuating mistruths, and we must couch our language in such a way that new myths are not created. The statement that "so-and-so had problems in school, too" is far more appropriate than a flat statement that "so-and-so had dyslexia just like you."

The scant evidence that has been presented has been usually based on an after-the-fact (or "after-life") diagnosis of the person's handwriting, and his reputed problems at school. But much more information than this is needed for an accurate diagnosis of dyslexia. In Chapter Nine concerning the possible causes of dyslexia, I mentioned the difficulty of adequately tracing dyslexia back three generations because of the problems of obtaining the necessary information to make a proper diagnosis of dyslexia. So too with these notable persons who lived a number of years ago and are reputed by some to have had dyslexia. Misspelled words, poor handwriting, and school problems do not necessarily add up to dyslexia! Yet a number of writers have made diagnoses on this basis.

Often there are more simple explanations for the difficulties these personages are said to have had. Pseudodyslexic symptoms may be caused by certain types of vision or hearing defects, inadequate or incorrect instruction in school, emotional problems, stress, anxiety, finger agnosia, or merely haste in writing in order to get thoughts down quickly on paper. Caution and careful investigation must be used—as well as plain common sense—in making any diagnosis, much less one based on historical assumptions.

Dr. Macdonald Critchley, neurologist, author of several books and many articles on dyslexia, who has studied more than 1,300 cases of dyslexia, characterizes the person who has been diagnosed as dyslexic at a young age, who has made progress while at school, and who has later embarked upon a career as follows:

> I suspect that he does not read for the sheer pleasure or fun of it like non-dyslexic individuals. He is not bookish; he doesn't browse in libraries like his contemporaries in age and intellectual attainment . . . [He] always continues to be a slow reader, so that it will take him an inordinate length of time to wade through a volume or a technical communication which would be skimmed through quite rapidly by a non-dyslexic. He is slow, furthermore, in getting the gist of a document or business statement, or quickly

identifying the nub of an argument or a legal brief. Maybe too, he is a somewhat inaccurate reader, and this may betray itself in his conversation. For example, he may consistently mispronounce certain words which are familiar enough to him from his reading, but which he does not associate with their spoken equivalents. The result is that in his conversation . . . [he] may make rather odd malapropisms when he comes to articulate words which are unusual or relatively infrequent in usage . . .

He is a most reluctant writer. In the same way he will be a slow writer and, I need scarcely say, an inaccurate speller. . . [There is] comparative brevity of [his] writings. Within a given unit of time, say thirty minutes [he] commits to paper far less materials than a non-dyslexic [and there is] a reduction of different words utilized. . . The dyslexic's writing is more monotonous. He does not employ particularly long sentences nor for that matter particularly short sentences. The average sentence length is intermediate and does not vary from sentence to sentence.

An important factor in writing is word-choice and word-usage. [He] rarely uses words of three or more syllables . . . will utilize an undue proportion of first person pronouns—I, me, we—which recur in his writings to an inordinate extent. Normal subjects are less personalized in their script and resort to far more abstract attitudes in the narrative. [The dyslexic] avoids utilizing abstract conceptions and is much more happy when he expresses on paper notions which are absolutely clear-cut, concrete, and identified with personal experience. [He is] very sparing of punctuation marks, and may limit himself solely to full stops. [One] would scarcely expect to find in [his] essays any foreign terms or expressions such as one might well come across in the prose of someone of comparable educational status and socio-cultural background.[1]

The above characteristics of dyslexics out of school and involved in careers are mentioned specifically in this chapter so that you can consider them as you read about the lives of certain persons described below. They are notable persons reputed to have been dyslexic. Among those most frequently cited are:

Hans Christian Andersen (Denmark's author of fairy tales)
King Charles XI of Sweden (Karl XI)
Winston Churchill (British prime minister during World War II)

Thomas Edison (American inventor)
Albert Einstein (renowned theoretical scientist, best known for his theory of relativity)
Leonardo da Vinci (Italian Renaissance artist)
George S. Patton, Jr. (American general in World War II)
Woodrow Wilson (twenty-eighth president of the United States)

These persons are no longer with us, of course, and they lived in times and places in which dyslexia was either unknown or little known. The diagnosis and remediation of dyslexia was certainly not part of a school's services. Any attempted diagnosis of dyslexia now, when these personages are no longer living, would have to rest purely upon speculation—risky business, surely for those who consider themselves professionals.

Let us briefly examine the lives of these men.

Hans Christian Andersen (1805–1875)

No one would deny that Hans Christian Andersen was the very talented, imaginative writer of many enchanting fairy tales. Less known is the fact that Andersen also wrote plays, novels, and travel books.

In respect to dyslexia, various points should be noted: effective stories must have an organized sequence of happenings; details in a tale, play, novel, or travel book are important; and visual imagery is essential for imaginative writing.

One source reported that Hans Christian Andersen only relatively recently has been discovered to have been a dyslexic, and this came about as the result of some "expert analysis" of his handwritten manuscripts.[2] Arriving at a diagnosis of dyslexia on the basis of handwriting alone is highly questionable. Spelling and handwriting errors may not be due to dyslexia at all but to a lot of reasons such as transposition and other reversal errors caused by finger agnosia, haste in getting racing ideas down on paper, stress—or just plain carelessness about spelling or handwriting. I do not read the words of the Danish language, but an examination of a reproduced sample of Andersen's handwriting did not show the numerous overwriting, erasures, and cross-overs so common to dyslexia. If they exist in other samples, they could still be caused by any of the reasons given above.

His misspelled words could easily be due to Andersen's inadequate education. One has to have the opportunity to learn to spell words. While Andersen did attend school for poor children in his hometown for a few years, he quit at age eleven after his father, a sickly, indigent shoemaker, died. Left alone entirely to his own devices, he built a toy theater and sat at home making clothes for his puppets—and, "avid reader" that he was, he read all the plays he could borrow, including those of Ludvig Holberg, father of Danish drama, and Shakespeare.[3,4]

When Andersen was fourteen years old he went to Copenhagen because he "was ambitious to become an opera singer,"[5] and he was befriended by the musicians Christoph Weyse and Siboni (and later by the poet Frederik Hoëgh Guldberg). When Andersen's voice failed to achieve his operatic ambitions, he was admitted as a dancing pupil at the Royal Theater.[6]

When he was seventeen years old he published his first book, *The Ghost at Palnatoke's Grave* (1822). He then was sent by his patron, King Frederick VI, to the grammar school at Slagelse. The king insisted that he remain there until he (the king) considered that Andersen was "educated." Andersen said that those five years were the darkest and bitterest in his life.[7]

But the assumption must not be made that his academic problems were due to dyslexia. It might well have been that his education at the Odense school for poor children had not prepared him for the performance expectations of the grammar school. The difference, moreover, in social background between the other students and Andersen may have embarrassed the sensitive young man. After having been on his own for six years, he may simply have found the rules and regulations of the school too restrictive.

At any rate, it is not likely that someone who possessed the vivid visual imagery and imagination of Andersen, the mastery of sequence, the ability to organize thoughts and set them down in stories, plays, and novels, and who willingly traveled on long journeys throughout Europe in order to write travel books the way Andersen did, would be a visual dyslexic. Nor is someone with operatic aspirations or who has been accepted in the Royal Theater dancing school likely to be an auditory dyslexic. Certainly a young dyslexic boy would not be considered an "avid reader," motivated to read on his own and to understand and enjoy plays by Ludvig Holberg and Shakespeare at age eleven. Andersen, moreover, enjoyed the acquaintance of Franz Liszt (the composer), Heinrich Heine (the poet), and Charles Dickens and Victor Hugo (the novelists), for they had interests in common.

Hans Christian Andersen surely was *not* a dyslexic.

King Charles XI (Karl XI) of Sweden (1655–1697)

King Charles XI may have had dyslexia. He apparently was a disappointing scholar, mainly because of his difficulty in learning to read. His progress in reading was extremely slow. As an adult he relied on personal interviews rather than on written reports—but many busy executives do this to save time. The difference lay here: if handed a paper, King Charles might hold it upside down and pretend to read it.[8] Could these problems be due to dyslexia? Could they be due instead to some kind of vision defect? This far removed in time we cannot know. We may never know.

His spelling is said to have been highly unconventional. He omitted letters in words, transposed letters (often starting with letters from the middle of the word), and reversed both letters and whole words. In an examination of his journals and other writings, Macdonald Critchley[9] discovered a number of interesting spelling mistakes, such as *ta* for *att* [transposition error plus omitted letter], *faton* for *aftou* [transposition error plus vertical reversal of *u* with *n*], *kråken* for *klockan* [blend and vowel confusions, plus silent letter omission], and *recyteran* for *rekryter* [letter substitution, blend error, letter omission, addition of letters at the end of the word]. Such spelling mistakes continued up to the time of King Charles' death.

But were these spelling mistakes due to reasons other than dyslexia, such as a vision defect? We cannot be sure at this late date. He certainly did have serious ongoing problems with reading and with writing, and it is possible that he had a combination of both visual and auditory dyslexia. All in all, "perhaps" is the word we should use if we wish to name King Charles XI as an example of a renowned dyslexic.

Winston Churchill (1874–1965)

Sir Winston Churchill was, among other things, an outstanding, spellbinding speaker, a noted historian and biographer, and a war reporter. He was a man of boundless energy with a vigorous mind. His command of the English language has been called "matchless," and he won the Nobel prize for literature in 1953.

Why is Churchill said to have had dyslexia? Probably because of his trouble with schoolwork, his refusal to learn Latin, and the fact that he spoke with a stutter as a child. (He also had a lisp.) As a boy his high spirits tended to get on everyone's nerves, and his stubborn nature and tenacity did not help the situation. His personality and strong will affected his schoolwork and antagonized his teachers. He worked hard for those masters he admired and respected—but not for those for whom he had no regard.

His speech problem must have been highly exasperating and frustrating to a boy with such a quick mind. On another front, his mother and father had many duties and responsibilities and could spare little time for their son. Trouble with schoolwork is one way to gain attention from parents. While we do not know that this was the case with Churchill, it is a possibility to be considered. The answer is more likely to lie in his competitiveness, his indifference to the authority of others, and his robust constitution. Only rarely did he play with other children, although he did enjoy football. His tastes, manners, recreation, and thinking reflected the adult world of politics in which he lived.[10]

Churchill's formal schooling began at Ascot, a fashionable and expensive institution. He ended up in the "caning room" frequently for "the headmaster was a sadist of a sort not uncommon in schools of that period, a man with whom flogging reached religious fervor. He felt that he was scourging out devils, and he sang at his work."[11] Such experiences were not likely to serve as a motivating educational force for a young boy of Churchill's nature. And it was here at Ascot that he refused to learn Latin. He viewed "the subject as a piece of calculated persecution on the part of the authorities."[12] Not learning Latin has been given as a reason to consider Churchill a dyslexic. But later, when he began writing speeches, he sat down and memorized a complete dictionary of Latin quotations![13] Here, too, at Ascot, he began writing a newspaper of his own, *The Critic*—not the type of task a dyslexic is likely to attempt.

While at Ascot Churchill read *King Solomon's Mines* by H. Rider Haggard. The young Churchill persuaded a relative of his to arrange a meeting with the author. Haggard came over and Winston quizzed him about various obscure passages in the book. "Now what do you mean by this business?" the child asked at one point, pointing to the passage in question. Haggard became very rattled and after reading the passage over, he admitted that he really did not have "the slightest idea."[14] This incident is not illustrative of typical dyslexia behavior and accomplishment.

When Churchill was twelve years old he entered a leading English secondary school, Harrow School, where it is said he got his love of the English language. With regard to dyslexia, I should mention Churchill's performance in qualifying in first place for Moriarty's Army Class. (Moriarty was the master who headed the Army Class and one whom Churchill especially admired.) While many boys of high scholastic standing failed this examination, Churchill had just learned 1,200 lines of Macaulay's "Lays of Ancient Rome" and recited them wihout a single error—again, not something a dyslexic is likely to be able to do.

For the army test Churchill knew that the contestants would be required to draw a map. The evening before he placed a collection of maps in his hat and then withdrew one, which turned out to be of New Zealand. He set about learning it. And Lady Luck was with the young Churchill, for he was asked to draw a map of New Zealand. His memory was in "well-oiled shape; he filled it in with such specificity including streams of a dozen yards' breadth and whistle stops on the narrow-gauge railroads, that Moriarty never quite got over it."[15] Again, such detail and such accuracy are not common to the visual dyslexic.

True, when it came time for Churchill to take the entrance examinations for the Royal Military College at Sandhurst (the English equivalent of the American West Point), he failed the examinations twice before passing them. This has been cited as part of the "proof" that Churchill had dyslexia. But never mentioned is the fact that he ended up *graduating eighth in a class of 150 students!* At Sandhurst he was particularly adept in tactics which involved fire and movement on the battlefield—finding ways of getting around the enemy. This, of course, required an adroitness in reading maps, a sense of organization and movement and direction in space, immediate recall, and the ability to shift one's thinking with quickness and clarity. Also, in the classrooms at Sandhurst, Churchill was "competent and quiet, in astonishing contrast to his classroom manner at Harrow." [16]

While stationed in Bangalore in southern India, Churchill read many of the books that he had neglected to read earlier. Among his favorites were the works of Edward Gibbon and Thomas B. Macaulay—certainly not the type of books that a dyslexic would select for pleasure reading, or be able to read at all.

A dyslexic has difficulty processing information quickly and setting his thoughts down in an organized fashion on paper. Winston Churchill was most adept at doing this and had no problems with details and sequence in his writings. He was a productive writer.

He also, quite obviously, had an excellent sense of direction. During the Boer War in South Africa when Churchill was riding on an armored train, the Boers ambushed the train and Churchill was captured. He escaped by scaling the prison wall and then crossed three hundred miles of enemy territory (in a country strange to him) by traveling on freight trains—a remarkable feat even for a nondyslexic.

One has only to listen to a record or tape of Sir Winston Churchill's speeches to be impressed with the fluency of his speech, his command of the language, and the orderliness, depth, speed and clarity of thought. He was famous as a master of repartee in parliamentary debates—his sharp mind and well-integrated speech flashed a quick retort at the propitious moment. He won the Nobel prize for "his mastery of historical and biographical presentation and for his brilliant oratory." [17]

Sir Winston Churchill was neither a visual nor an auditory dyslexic.

Thomas Alva Edison (1847–1931)

Thomas A. Edison had a phenomenal mind, endless curiosity, an abundance of energy, tremendous initiative and drive, and enormous "stick-to-it-ive-ness." What he accomplished in his lifetime is incredible. He was certainly one of the great technical geniuses in history. His inventions include an electric vote-recording machine, a typewriter that later became the Remington, the quadruple telegraph repeaters for simultaneous dispatch of several messages over a single wire, the phonograph, the incandescent electric lamp, the electric dynamo, the mimeograph machine, the motion picture camera, the transmitter, and others too numerous to list.

In proof that Edison had dyslexia, the evidence given was that he was considered a dunce at school, that he could not learn the alphabet or arithmetic tables by heart, and that his spelling and grammar remained poor throughout his life. [18,19] Yet the truth of the matter is that because of his need to know the "why" of things, his tenacity in asking questions, he remained in public school for *only three months*. It seems that Edison irritated his schoolmaster by asking too many questions. When Edison overheard his teacher refer to him as "addled," he told his mother, a former schoolteacher herself. She immediately confronted the schoolmaster and told him that her son had more sense in his little finger than the schoolmaster had in his entire body (which Edison probably did have)—and she withdrew Thomas from school and set about teaching him at home.

Edison's mother believed that learning did not have to be drudgery but could and should be fun. Edison was enchanted with this approach and progressed so rapidly that his mother could no longer instruct him. He was not a "dunce" at all, nor "addled." Indeed, Edison read a chemistry book (by Richard G. Parker) with such understanding that he questioned certain statements made by the author—and set about proving them incorrect. Hardly something a dyslexic boy would do.

When he was sixteen, Edison became a telegrapher—another task difficult for a dyslexic because of the coding and sound patterns, sequencing, and need for memory and immediate recall. He was supposed to check in with the Toronto office every hour by telegraph signal. This was a nuisance, so the ingenious Edison constructed a means of sending the hourly signal by attaching a gadget to a clock. Edison lost several jobs because of his fondness for reading and his boredom with routine, uncreative work. He read intensely throughout his life. When on the path of inventing something, his procedure would be *to seclude himself for days reading everything he could get his hands on concerning the topic*, not only from his vast library next to his laboratory, but from whatever his literary agent could obtain. Only then, after a thorough review of the subject, would he begin his laboratory work. By doing this he avoided the failures of others as well as the fruitless repetition of old experiments.[20]

Thomas Alva Edison a dyslexic? Hardly. A nine-year-old dyslexic is not likely to read a chemistry book at all, much less with such understanding, nor have a fondness for reading in general as did Edison. Learning and using the Morse code would be next to impossible. Scientific experiments require very careful, methodical steps and organized thinking, and an ability to focus on a task for long periods. Dyslexics are not likely to immerse themselves in a variety of books on a particular topic for days and days at a time. The evidence does *not* support the notion that Edison was a dyslexic.

Albert Einstein (1879–1955)

Einstein is probably the most often cited "dyslexic" in the books and articles on dyslexia. But, as Macdonald and Eileen Critchley point out in their book, *Dyslexia Defined*, "the evidence for Einstein being a true case . . . is slight.[21] They do not elaborate upon this statement.

What is the evidence for Einstein's being dyslexic? The following is offered by several writers. Einstein did not talk until he was three years old nor read until he was nine.[22,23] There was evidence of frustration in Einstein's early education, such as when at age five, during a session with his special tutor for lessons and music, it seems that he became so upset that he threw a chair at his teacher who left, never to return. He was a fair-to-middling student in the early school years, (but by the age of twelve he was a brilliant mathematician and physicist). He had no gift for languages. He failed his language requirement at the public school in Munich and left at age fifteen without a diploma. He also failed the language requirements for admission to technical school and enrolled in a small canton school where there was a minimum of verbal communication and a maximum use of diagrams, maps, and charts, as well as demonstration.[24]

What is the meaning of this "evidence"? It is not unusual for some highly intelligent children to delay their speaking, but when they do speak they tend to speak in complete sentences, rather than speaking one or two words in isolation. Age five, furthermore, is early to begin formal lessons. We know nothing about the teacher's relationship with Einstein nor the teaching techniques used nor performance expectations for the child. The temper tantrum could well have been the result of a young five-year-old from whom too much was expected too soon. Intellectually gifted children can be mediocre students for one reason or another, especially if they are creative and are expected to conform, and if they are bored in class. As far as the language requirements are concerned, Einstein's interests quite obviously lay in other directions. As an adult, he could speak and write in English in addition to his native German.

Visual dyslexia? One of the sources reported that Einstein was unusually adept at working puzzles, including geometric puzzles—before the age of ten! And he read, marked, and annotated a geometry book at age twelve.[25] Using diagrams, charts, and maps requires visual memory. His unique ability to grasp concepts of space, mass, motion, time, and gravitation at any level is nigh miraculous—indeed, he changed the way we think about things. Einstein wrote about these concepts with clarity, preciseness, and orderliness. The development of his different theories required exact steps in sequence and clearness of thought.

Auditory dyslexia? Einstein was very fond of classical music and enjoyed playing the violin, neither of which is probable with auditory dyslexia. He also spoke and wrote in English, a difficult language to learn, so it is said.

The verdict? It is exceedingly doubtful that Einstein was a dyslexic, either visual or auditory, and he should not be cited as such. The publication of children's books, such as *Einstein and Me* (about a dyslexic boy who attends Einstein School, and in which Einstein is referred to as a dyslexic), should be discouraged.

Leonardo da Vinci (1452–1519)

Leonardo da Vinci is often reported as having been a dyslexic, yet he was a painter, sculptor, musician, architect, experimental scientist, military engineer, art critic, and fiction writer! His figures, portraits, and designs were true to life, exceptionally realistic; these required a strong visual memory, an eye for detail, a sense of direction, a sureness of touch. Architectural drawings are like maps and charts and require a high level of accuracy in planning and execution, and a strong perception of direction, size, and space.

Leonardo was a lute player and had a beautiful voice. He studied the physics of music and understood the fundamentals of acoustics and the physics of the echo.[26]

He had a country schoolboy's education. "He grumbled at not having Latin and Greek," writes Richie Calder in his biography of Leonardo, "but he set out to teach himself, just as he taught himself, quite effectively, advanced forms of mathematics to the level where he would vaunt 'Let no man who is not a mathematician read the elements of my work'—echoing Plato who inscribed over the entrance to his Academy 'Let no one ignorant of geometry enter here.' Leonardo had a natural curiosity and a thirst for knowledge of all things which were not discouraged by his early schooldays.[27]

"Apart from his uncommon 'common sense' " Calder goes on—"the brain, the recipient sense common to all physical senses, his faculties, certainly those of sight and hearing, were exceptionally acute . . . His color register [discrimination] was similarly exceptional not just in seeing the obvious colour differences in painting, but in the subtlety of hues which he expressed in his theory of colours . . . His [hearing] sensitivity suggests a range and a precision which was not really available scientifically until we had the microphone and high-fidelity recordings, and the cathode ray oscillograph to make sound visible . . . He was lucky to be apprenticed to Verrocchio at a time when perspective had become a preoccupation of artists. This at its simplest was the geometry of drawing . . . Leonardo could encompass, as well as create, the knowledge of his times. He was exceptional in his perceptions and his breadth of awareness. No single man today could embrace all the knowledge of all the disciplines which he embodied . . . He relied upon his senses, but was always insistent that the senses were the servants of 'the common sense,' the brain."[28]

Leonardo had such a keen intellect that he acquired information with little effort. He studied geometry and physics and astronomy and anatomy and physiology *on his own*. He was a renowned inventor. Among his numerous inventions were the free-moving ball bearing, needle-sharpening machine, chimney cowl to divert smoke, diving suit, military tank, sliding ladder, machine gun, oil lamp, and swing bridge. He was a successful engineer, and "perhaps the deepest thinker and most profound investigator into all the known branches of science of his age." [29]

Leonardo da Vinci wrote *Treatise on Painting*, intended as a guide and mentor for his own pupils and as a reflection on his own work as well as that of other artists. He kept voluminous notes, and there are today almost seven thousand pages remaining, containing comments, notes, sketches, and his philosophy of life.

He was ambidextrous, able to use both hands equally well in writing. *He read and wrote competently in the conventional forms.* On his sketches he wrote special notes for himself *in Latin* with his left hand, in a right to left direction from the margin. He created his own style of shorthand—grammalogues, combining words and phrases and using symbols.[30,31,32]

Some historians claim that he wrote in this manner deliberately so as to disguise his thoughts and protect his inventions. But, unfortunately someone saw these unique notes on Leonardo's sketches and rushed to the conclusion that he was dyslexic because of his "mirror-writing," without investigating the situation further. And thus, was birth given to the myth that Leonardo da Vinci was a dyslexic.

Understanding of true "mirror-writing" is limited, and any explanation of this phenomenon is highly speculative.[33,34] But one can be certain that da Vinci did not suffer from the spatial, orientation, and directional confusions that usually cause mirror-writing. Leonardo was simply a genius, a gifted artist who created his own special form of shorthand for his own particular purposes. As already mentioned, he could write quite proficiently in the conventional manner. It is ludicrous to use Leonardo da Vinci as an example of a famous dyslexic.

George S. Patton, Jr. (1885–1945)

Now the general's name is being thrown into the collective basket of notable dyslexics. One source reports that Patton could not read well although he had a fantastic "verbal memory." And he had to have someone write down his examination answers for him.[35] Another writes that "he got through West Point by memorizing whole lectures and texts and parroting them verbatim." [36]

What are the facts in the case of Patton? In the early years, Patton did not have to go to school. His father did not believe in formal education for his children, although he was a cultured man of wide knowledge gained by study and reading. He believed that young brains were unduly burdened with the strict stereotyped curricula of schools, especially the three R's—reading, 'riting and 'rithmetic. He preferred to impart whatever education he thought they needed by reading the classics to them on long evenings in front of their huge fireplace. By the time he was seven years old, George Patton could recite long passages from the *Illiad* in Pope's translation and knew much of the Bible by heart.[37] Ask yourself, is this something that a seven-year-old dyslexic would be able to do?

When Patton was twelve years old his father decided to begin his formal education. Patton could neither read nor write—not because he was dyslexic but because he had never been taught! He could recite long passages (with the sequencing correct), but he could not put them down on paper. Yet "Georgie quickly managed to learn to read and became an accomplished writer—as shown by the many brilliant articles which he contributed to the old *Cavalry Journal*; by the facile style of his diary; the lucid notes in his *War As I Knew It*; his letters to his wife—and especially by his crisp and highly professional instructions and orders to his troops." [38]

True, Patton never did learn to spell well, and he was weak in arithmetic. But why just assume that this was due to dyslexia? He missed all those early years of schooling when a stock of spelling words and the basic math facts are acquired. We do not know whether Dr. Stephen Cotter Clark's Classical School for Boys gave individual attention to these deficiencies.

Patton went on to graduate from Pasadena High School, spent a year at the Virginia Military Institute, and passed the entrance examinations for West Point. (I have found no mention of the West Point examinations answers being written by someone else. At any rate, it is doubtful that this would have been allowed.) He did flunk his math test in his plebe year at West Point. The reason for this may be because he had been trained by his father to memorize "everything verbatim" and he found the problems in Smith's *Algebra* very difficult.[39] But he read avidly whatever books he could find dealing with military history.[40] He read in depth and retained the information to the minutest detail. His recall, even years later, was remarkable as to time, detail, sequence, movement, direction, location, space, number, and action. Map reading, topographical features of the terrain, flexibility and change in direction gave him no problems.

Patton's difficulties were likely due to his lack of formal education in those early years, rather than to dyslexia. I would not include him in any list of dyslexics.

Woodrow Wilson (1856–1924)

Another name recently added to the "dyslexia file" is that of Woodrow Wilson, twenty-eighth president of the United States. He was a professor of history, president of Princeton University, a political leader, and a popular and

163

distinguished lecturer and writer. He had a great deal of energy, a magnetic personality, and a fantastic mind.

He graduated from Princeton University thirty-eighth in a class of 106. While there he practiced public speaking, was a leader in debating, and read widely on public affairs; and he was managing editor of the college newspaper. He then entered law school at the University of Virginia where he was active in the debating societies. He was an outstanding student at UVA but ill health forced him to leave the following winter.

After a brief interlude as a practicing lawyer, Wilson wanted to be a college teacher and did graduate work at Johns Hopkins where he received his Ph.D. degree in 1886.

Wilson was a family man, an avid reader, and spent many evenings with his three daughters telling stories and reading aloud from Dickens, Wordsworth, and Scott. He wrote a number of books including *The State, Congressional Government* (his doctoral dissertation), *Division and Reunion, Constitutional Government, A History of the American People* (five volumes), *George Washington*, and *The New Freedom* (his campaign speeches).

Some of the "evidence" given for citing Wilson as being dyslexic is based on his handwriting.[41] Wilson felt the frustration and stress of being unable to write his thoughts down fast enough to keep up with his quick, active mind—so he taught himself shorthand. Learning these symbols would be difficult for a true dyslexic under any circumstances, and it is unlikely a dyslexic would teach them to himself. Anyone who has learned shorthand knows that some of these symbols tend to creep into ordinary handwriting when one has to write something in a hurry.

Wilson turned to the typewriter no doubt for the same reason many other writers do—to keep up with a fast-moving, creative mind so that the flow of thoughts will continue with no interruption in fluency.

Wilson, at age seventeen, had attended a year at Davidson. He had been poorly prepared for college. He had been conditioned in Cicero and in ancient geography by his father, but he entered his Greek and mathematics classes on probation, and he was required to make up a heavy amount of back work. His report card for the first term was as follows: [42,43]

Composition and English 96
Logic and Rhetoric.. 95
Declamation [oratory].. 92
Latin 90
Greek.. 87
Mathematics.. 74
Deportment..100

For the second term report, his grades were: [44]

English... 97
Composition.. 95
Latin 94
Declamation 92
Greek.. 88
Mathematics.. 88
Deportment..100

As shown here, Wilson's highest grades were in composition and English, the lowest in mathematics and Greek. But these grades in these subjects, including Latin and Greek, could not be called typical of courses taken by and grades won by any young seventeen-year-old dyslexic. (Interestingly, some writers have used difficulties in foreign language as symptomatic of dyslexia, yet Wilson did quite well in both Latin and Greek, and also mastered German and French—but the critics seem to have overlooked this fact.)

Several sources reported that Wilson was dyslexic because "he did not learn his letters until nine" or learn to read until he was eleven.[45,46,47] But the truth of the matter is that Wilson did not even start school until he was nine years old because the Civil War had closed so many of them.[48] One of Wilson's biographers mentions that "he did not even learn his letters until he was nine years old; and could not read readily until he was eleven," *but the biographer went on to add*, "What need was there when a boy could spend eight hours in delightful listening while others read aloud? [His father and sisters read aloud to him frequently.] He loved always the spoken word, the roll of language." [49] The process of reading is complex, and two years would be a normal time for a bright child to begin reading "readily" from the time of first learning his alphabet letters. It is worth speculating that Wilson, an eminent man of letters, may actually have had an advantage in not being forced to learn to read at too early an age!

While Wilson's father taught him a great deal at home, his grandfather, who was a frequent visitor and a devotee of the ancient classics, also contributed substantially to Wilson's training. The young Wilson made short trips with his father, after which the boy would be encouraged to relate what he had seen. His father stressed that an exact expression of ideas was essential for clear understanding. This the young boy was able to do competently.

One of Wilson's main interests when he was a youngster was a club which he organized himself. The members played baseball, challenging the neighborhood teams. While Wilson was not the best player, he was president of the club and he wrote a constitution for it before he was ten years old. Rules of strict parliamentary procedure governed all debates of the club members![50] These are not likely activities for a ten-year-old dyslexic.

One of Wilson's classmates at Davidson spoke of him as a "fine, graceful young man, brilliant in his studies and as an athlete. As a short stop on the college team he was a handy player." At Princeton he sang in the Glee Club, was president of the Athletic Committee, and president of the Baseball Association. He made "deep friendships that were never broken."[51] Another biographer stated that "as in his student days, he formed strong friendships . . . Every Sunday afternoon for years an intimate little group met . . . for tea and hours of animated talk."[52] Yet Woodrow Wilson has been described as being "a loner," and this given as evidence of his dyslexia![53]

You will recall, as quoted at the beginning of this chapter, that adult dyslexics are "slow . . . identifying the nub of an argument or legal brief." Wilson was admitted to the bar in 1885.[54]

An examination of Wilson's speeches and writings and a study of his life reveal a clarity and fluency of thought, skillful manipulation of details and organization of facts, excellent recall, and a zest for reading and the acquisition of knowledge.

> All his life he had been a reader: no casual reader, but one of the eager and passionate kind who is not content until he tears out the very heart of a book. This was true not only of so-called serious books, but of romances and poetry as well. When the boy read Cooper's novels, he wished afterward to act them out; if he read sea stories, he made pictures of the ships described; and he was not content with Scott's romances until he had found someone— his father was his best resource—with whom he could discuss the characters and incidents. Many of the volumes of his reading remained in his library at his death. They are indicative of his passion to know completely and accurately what the author had to say. Here, for example, are such books as *The Federalist*, Green's *Short History of the English People*—and Macaulay and Bagehot—with the pages underscored and marginally noted to the last degree, and often written synopses appended to the chapter."[55]

In a commendable effort to dispel one myth about Woodrow Wilson, i.e., Freudian interpretations for a number of things, two researchers (an educational psychologist and a historian)[56] have fallen into the trap of perpetuating another myth—that Wilson had dyslexia. They even threaten to publish a whole volume on historic persons who allegedly, on highly questionable grounds, have had dyslexia.[57]

Woodrow Wilson a dyslexic? Balderdash! The facts do not support this notion, and this myth should not continue to be fostered.

* * * * * * * *

Others Reputed to Have Been Dyslexic

There are other notable persons less frequently cited as having been dyslexic. Some of these are: Harvey Cushing (the pioneer in brain surgery[58] and a prolific writer, who won the Pulitzer prize in biography for his book, *The Life of Sir William Osler*); Paul Ehrlich (the German bacteriologist and discoverer of the drug to destroy the specific organism of syphilis); David Lloyd George (British prime minister during World War I); William James (American philosopher and psychologist who wrote philosophy in a wonderfully readable style); Abbott Lawrence Lowell (former president of Harvard University); Michelangelo (the Italian Renaissance artist); and Auguste Rodin (the French sculptor).

As in the case of the persons discussed in more detail earlier, an examination of these men's lives and their works and a search for plausible explanations for certain academic problems raise serious doubts about labeling any as dyslexic. It is highly improbable that they were, and they should not be cited as such in view of the insufficient evidence proffered.

The Credibility Gap

If we are ever to achieve a cooperative, interdisciplinary approach to the dyslexia problem, we who work with dyslexics must earn the respect of those in the various disciplines. Perhaps the credibility gap that now exists is partly due to a few well-meaning persons who have been eager to bring about acceptance of the dyslexia concept and have been too eager to reassure dyslexics and parents by citing as dyslexics persons of substantial accomplishments. Of course we want dyslexics and their parents to feel good about themselves and to hope for a brighter future, but hope must have a firmer basis than quoting myths.

In some cases, this mythologizing has produced ludicrous results. I know of instances where parents will insist that a child is dyslexic, though there are other causes for the problems, because for them the term, dyslexia, has become some kind of status symbol—look at all the famous intellects who have had it, they crow. For some who cannot accept the real reasons for their children's problems, dyslexia is a comforting explanation.

Those of us in the professional fields must keep our feet on the ground, always using a common-sensible, professional approach in these matters. Diagnosis should never be made on the basis of a few symptoms and insufficient information. We need to search for all possible reasons behind a problem and consider the facts objectively. For example, if a sample of mirror-writing is uncovered, one does not immediately jump to the conclusion that a person is dyslexic. Teachers and others who need to explain things are sometimes placed in situations where they must write backward on a glass, allowing a viewer on the opposite side to read the information. Technicians and non-commissioned officers in the military services write backward on glass charts. Merchants write backward on display windows. Television weathermen sometimes write backward on the glass weather chart. Left-handed children in the early grades seem to have a natural tendency to begin writing from right to left.

I can remember as a child exchanging secret letters with friends which were written backward and later we would hold these up to a mirror so we could more easily read what was written. (Would someone finding one of these letters tucked away in the attic conclude that we were dyslexic?)

Of course, one must always consider the possibility that a printer at one time or another may have simply reversed the negatives of an illustration or made typographical errors. Some Shakespearean "purists" still get very upset if certain words are changed in his works—some of which are the result, not of Shakespeare's writing, but of a printer's error.

Most people will occasionally transpose letters when dialing a telephone number, especially when in a hurry. What typist has not transposed letters when typing—again especially when in a hurry or under stress? Who has not transposed letters in simple words when writing letters? These errors tend to occur also when the people do not have their mind on what they are doing or when in a hurry or under stress. Just plain carelessness is probably the number one culprit of errors in spelling. Diagnosing dyslexia on the evidence of a person's writing alone is altogether unreliable.

But what if there are many such errors? What then? Again, caution is advised. Look to the schooling of the person. Did he have the *opportunity* to learn? What about his personality? Was he the type of person who would place a priority on correct spelling—or were other things more important, such as getting down his ideas quickly any way he could?

What about his reading? Did he read early and widely? What types of books did he read? Was he an excellent reader but a careless speller? Could he set his ideas down in written form in an organized, sequential manner? Was he a fluent speaker expressing himself with clarity and conciseness and orderliness? Did he enjoy music? Play a musical instrument? Sing in the choir? A good dancer?

In sum, it should be remembered that (1) in any diagnosis of dyslexia the whole person must be considered—his background, his opportunity to learn, what he has accomplished in various areas, his personality, (2) diagnosis cannot be made on any single factor, and (3) any retroactive diagnosis, as in these cases, is highly precarious.

* * * * * * *

Obviously none of the notable persons cited in this chapter had access to any program for diagnosing and remediating dyslexia. If the purpose of perpetuating the myth of their dyslexia is to reassure dyslexic children and their parents, the essence of the message is actually: "You do not need to do anything. You do not need to see a reading specialist or a learning disability teacher for regular remediation of your dyslexia condition. It will go away with time. In fact, you are likely to be a far greater achiever than the so-called normal persons."

Nonsense!

Notes for Chapter 12

1. Macdonald Critchley, "Some Problems of the Ex-Dyslexic," *Bulletin of the Orton Society* 23 (1973), pp. 9–13. Used with permission.
2. Bevé Hornsby *Overcoming Dyslexia* (New York: Arco, 1984), p. 12.
3. "Andersen, Hans Christian," *The Encyclopedia Americana* Vol. 1 (1946), p. 658.
4. Edmund Gosse, "Andersen, Hans Christian," *The Encyclopedia Brittannica*, 11th ed., Vol. 1 (1911), p. 958.
5. "Andersen, Hans Christian," *The Encyclopedia Americana* Vol. 1 (1946), p. 658.
6. Gosse, op.cit., p. 958.
7. Ibid.
8. Macdonald Critchley, *The Dyslexic Child* (Springfield, Ill.: Charles C. Thomas, 1970), p. 114.
9. Ibid., pp. 114–115.
10. Robert Lewis Taylor, *Winston Churchill, An Informal Study of Greatness* (Garden City, New York: Doubleday, 1952), p. 47.
11. Ibid., pp. 53, 55.
12. Ibid., p. 54.
13. Ibid.
14. Ibid., pp. 58–59.
15. Ibid., pp. 70–71.
16. Ibid., p. 91.
17. Carol L. Thompson, "Churchill, Sir Winston Leonard Spencer," *The World Book Encyclopedia* Vol. 3 (1969), p. 425.

18. Hornsby, op.cit., p. 12
19. Lloyd J. Thompson, "Language Disabilities in Men of Eminence," *Journal of Learning Disabilities* Vol. 4 (January 1971), pp. 39–44.
20. "Edison, Thomas Alva," *The Encyclopedia Americana* Vol. 9 (1946), p. 588.
21. Macdonald Critchley and Eileen Critchley, *Dyslexia Defined* (Springfield, Ill.: Charles C. Thomas, 1978), p. 133.
22. Hornsby, op.cit., p. 10.
23. Thompson, op.cit., p. 116.
24. Richard L. Masland, "The Advantages of Being Dyslexic," *Bulletin of the Orton Society* Vol. 26 (1976), pp. 15–17.
25. Ibid., p. 17.
26. Richie Calder, *Leonardo and the Age of the Eye* (New York: Simon and Schuster, 1970), p. 87.
27. Ibid., p. 260.
28. Ibid., pp. 260–261, 273–274.
29. "Vinci, Leonardo da," *The Encyclopedia Americana* Vol. 28 (1946), p. 100.
30. Raymond S. Stites, "Da Vinci, Leonardo," *The World Book Encyclopedia* Vol. 5 (1969), p. 41.
31. Sidney Colvin, "Leonardo da Vinci," *Encyclopedia Britannica* 11th ed., Vol. 16 (1911), p. 453.
32. Calder, op.cit., p. 36.
33. Frank R. Vellutino, *Dyslexia: Theory and Research* (Cambridge, Mass.: The MIT Press, 1979), p. 137.
34. Note on mirror-writing: Mirror-writing does not make one a dyslexic. I have observed that when young children first learn to write they will sometimes begin to write from the right margin to the left. The problem can be simply solved by marking the left side of the paper, or placing a watch or ring on the left hand, and calling the child's attention to this. Usually it can be solved by simply telling a left-handed child to begin starting at the edge of the page on the same side as the hand he uses for writing. The right-handed child is told to start on the side across from his "writing hand." I have noticed that lefties tend to be more persistent in this behavior. For older students who have not had the difficulty firmly corrected and have had insufficient left-to-right orientation practice, I have found this procedure plus tracing techniques (a line of writing) has worked quite successfully. Indeed, as far back as 1943, Grace Fernald reports on correcting an eleven-year-old's mirror-writing in a period of only five days by these simple methods. Grace Gernald, *Remedial Techniques in Basic School Subjects* (New York: McGraw-Hill, 1943), pp. 90–91.
35. Hornsby, op.cit., p. 12.
36. Thompson, op.cit., p. 116.
37. Ladislas Farago, *Patton: Ordeal and Triumph* (New York: Dell, 1963), pp. 55–56.
38. Ibid., p. 56.
39. Ibid., pp. 56, 57–58.
40. Ibid., p. 45.

41. Mary Wade Atteberry, "Dyslexia, Do Its Victims Have Unusual Ability?" *The Indianapolis Star* Section F (Nov. 4, 1984), pp. 1–2.
42. Ray Stannard Baker, *Woodrow Wilson, Life and Letters; Youth 1856–1890* (New York: Doubleday, 1927), pp. 74–75.
43. Ruth Cranston, *The Story of Woodrow Wilson* (New York: Simon and Schuster, 1945), pp. 15–16.
44. Baker, op.cit., p. 74.
45. Hornsby, op.cit., p. 12.
46. Thompson, op.cit., p. 116.
47. Elizabeth Fleming, *Believe the Heart* (San Francisco, Calif.: Strawberry Hill, 1984), p. 39.
48. Arthur S. Link, "Wilson, Woodrow," *The World Book Encyclopedia* Vol. 20 (1969), p. 269.
49. Baker, op.cit., p. 36.
50. Cranston, op.cit., pp. 8–9; Baker, op.cit., p. 45.
51. Josephus Daniels, *The Life of Woodrow Wilson* (Chicago: John C. Winston, 1924), p. 43, 48, 58.
52. Cranston, op.cit., p. 53.
53. Atteberry, op.cit., p. 2.
54. Arthur S. Link, *Wilson, The Road to the White House* (Princeton, New Jersey: Princeton University, 1947), p. 8.
55. Baker, op.cit., p. 86.
56. P. G. Aaron and Robert G. Clouse at Indiana State University.
57. Atteberry, op.cit., p. 2.
58. Cushing was a noted brain surgeon at Johns Hopkins, Harvard and Yale. How would you feel about having a dyslexic with problems in sequence and left/right, up/down, in/out concepts and directions operate on you or your loved ones? Obviously Cushing did not have that kind of difficulty.

PART FIVE: WHAT CAN WE DO ABOUT IT?

Nothing in education is so astonishing
as the amount of ignorance it accumulates
in the form of inert facts.

—*Henry Adams*

CHAPTER

13

ALLEVIATING DYSLEXIA

Nothing can be taught unless it has the
potential of making sense to the learner, and
learning itself is nothing but the endeavor
to make sense. The effort to teach or to
inform, therefore, can be nothing but an
endeavour to make sense, to be
comprehensible.

—Frank Smith

If a child has visual dyslexia, it can generally be more readily alleviated and in less time than auditory dyslexia. This statement, however, should not be taken to imply that visual dyslexia always can be very quickly remediated, nor that auditory dyslexia is beyond help. The length of time for the alleviation of any type of dyslexia depends upon several factors:

The severity of the dyslexia
The intelligence of the dyslexic student
The willingness of the student to work
The age of the dyslexic
The expertise of the person alleviating the dyslexia
The materials available in the classroom and clinic

The cooperation and understanding of the parents
The cooperation and understanding of the classroom teacher
The duration and frequency of periods, and length of remediation
Whether the remediation is on a one-to-one basis or in a small group
situation

The Severity of the Problem

I have found that the dyslexic condition can range from severe to moderate to mild. Just as when a child has a physical illness such as pneumonia, the more severely ill a child is, the longer the recovery. The milder the case of pneumonia, the more quickly the child snaps back. So, too, with dyslexia.

The Intelligence of the Dyslexic Student

Intelligence is a major factor in learning and progressing in school. The more intelligent student tends to pick up new concepts and vocabulary more quickly and to learn at a faster rate. Retention of material learned is better. The slow learning child needs much more repetition and review. There is less retention; hence the need for additional repetition and review which takes more time. These differences have added significance for the dyslexic.

The Willingness of the Student to Work

The willingness of the dyslexic to work is no doubt just as important as intelligence, for no matter how intelligent a student may be, if he is not motivated and does not want to work and to learn—he won't. In remediation, as in all education, the sixty-four dollar question for teachers becomes, "How can I motivate this child, get him interested in learning?"

A dyslexic who has been having problems in school—given work which he cannot do and then reprimanded by the teacher for not doing it—who has received low grades for which he has been chastised by his parents, who has become aware that he cannot do the same work as his classmates, and who has been kept in at recess and sometimes after school to complete work which is frustrating to him—this child is not likely to continue to have that natural curiosity and zest for learning that are a natural part of any child and which he brings with him when he enters school.

What happens? He will be afraid to try, to take a chance on making a mistake, for he is fearful of failure, fearful of ridicule, fearful of seeing red marks all over his papers with the customary low grade written at the top or having comments by the teacher such as, "You can do better if you only try," or "Pay attention in class. You should have learned this material."

But these students *can* be motivated. They *can* become excited about learning and progressing. In the clinic, we find that in the first week of attendance, the children are inclined to be somewhat on the defensive, sometimes putting on a facade of not caring about anything. But as time goes on, and they

176

find themselves in a secure environment of trust and faith that they can learn, find out they are not really "dumb," see they are learning each day, get work and materials of particular interest to them, receive frequent encouragement and praise—then they become willing to take another chance, to try to learn even though they might be wrong . . . and then to try again.

Learning takes initiative and drive, but these do not automatically occur in a classroom nor in a child who has had repeated failures. The child must be nourished. Those around him must trust in his ability to learn. They must be able to "turn him on" so that he will be willing to try, willing to work hard. Successful teaching results in a bond between the teacher and the student. Each becomes inspired by and inspiring to the other. Both become learners in this process.

The Age of the Dyslexic

The longer a child is ill, the more worn down he becomes and consequently the longer his recovery. The older the dyslexic child (beyond the age of eight or nine, of course), the longer he has endured failure and frustration, the lower his self-esteem—how he sees himself and how he perceives that others in his world view him. He has had to learn all kinds of coping and survival techniques to make it in school and at home. Negative behaviors, reenforced over and over, have become habitual.

The older the dyslexic is, the farther behind he has fallen in his school work. He may have had to repeat one or more grades, and he is embarrassed and humiliated as his friends leave him behind and move on up to higher grades. He may truly believe that he is stupid. He may have arrived at the point of desperation: "What's the use of trying?" Such negative concepts have to be eliminated, of course, before remediation can become effective.

The following statement is especially appropriate in dealing with a dyslexic student:

> Every time we succeed at something which is important to us, we make a deposit in our emotional bank account. Each time we are diminished by something someone does or says, we make a withdrawal. Some people, some children, are always in the red, always overdrawn.[1]

I have found that the older a dyslexic student is, the more overdrawn his emotional bank account.

The Expertise of the Person Alleviating the Dyslexia

The knowledge, training, understanding, and experience of the person working with the dyslexic student will affect the progress of the remediation. What good does it do to diagnose dyslexia, pinpoint specifically the deficiencies of the dyslexic, and then send him to someone for remediation who does not know what to do about alleviating the various problems?

Ignorance on the part of this person can in fact compound the problem and even create new problems where none existed before. In some college and university programs, graduate students are required to take diagnostic courses, but not a remediation course for disabilities. Other schools of education offer a one-semester course combining both diagnosis and remediation, with the result that diagnosis usually gets the major emphasis. In any case, in the latter situation the students tend to get too much information too fast—not enough time to absorb and retain the necessary knowledge to be proficient in both diagnosis and remediation.

A competent person who knows exactly what to do to alleviate dyslexia and how to do it can accomplish a great deal in a reasonable length of time. Do these troubled young dyslexics deserve any less than the best? They have already paid the price.

The Materials Available in the Classroom and Clinic

All too often administrators, rather than teachers, decide what materials to order and then tell the teachers to do the job without their having the appropriate tools to do it effectively. This can be frustrating to even the most capable and conscientious of teachers. How can a mechanic possibly make repairs to the engine of a car without the proper tools for the job? How can a surgeon possibly operate without the necessary medical instruments to perform the operation? There are tools that teachers need in order to teach interesting and creative lessons that will result in successful learning on the part of students. These tools are the materials available in the classroom to help get the job of teaching done.

I am not talking about tables full of basal reader workbooks, multiple phonics workbooks, stacks of purple dittoed skill sheets, or various commercial "cookbook" programs. This type of material too often becomes a crutch for lazy or ill-prepared teachers. Too frequently such materials end up determining the remediation program. No, I am referring to quantities of books at various levels of difficulty and on different topics which would be of interest to the individual student. I am referring to materials that would not insult nor humiliate the more mature student. The older dyslexic student who may be reading at the preprimer, primer, or first grade level is embarrassed to have to read something like, "The duck says quack, quack, quack. Come here, duck. Come here, duck. Can you say quack, quack, quack?" There are books available that do not have the appearance of "baby books"; they have smaller type, the lines of print are closer together, and they have illustrations of older children rather than first-graders. (Listed in Appendix C are the names and addresses of publishers of "high-interest, low vocabulary" books designed for use in remediation of older students not reading on grade level.)

Teachers will need plenty of chart paper for experience charts and practical charts for teaching new words, and sentence strips and pocket charts for teaching new vocabulary and developing sequencing. They also need construction paper, paste, scissors, magic markers, crayons, string, blocks, puzzles, sand and glue for preparing kinesthetic tracing materials, wooden letters in both capitals and lower case, dolls and clothing, boxes and cans from the grocery store, and boxes and cards for the students' word banks.

For older students, materials should include driver's license manuals, hunting and fishing pamphlets, magazines about such sports as tennis, swimming, skating, surfing, hockey, baseball, football, basketball, and soccer, and books and magazines about airplanes, racing cars, motorbikes, and bicycles. There should be cookbooks; Cub Scout, Brownie, Boy Scout, and Girl Scout books; clothing and fashion magazines; telephone books; travel guidebooks; maps of the city, county, state, the United States and the world; TV Guides, and other popular magazines—even a few comic books.

Magazines and books such as these can be used for application of all kinds of learning. One does not need a phonics workbook to teach phonics; any of the above will do! New words, sequencing skills, dividing words into syllables—and many other items and skills—can be taught by using common materials.

Spending day after day filling in the blanks on workbook pages or dittoed sheets, keeping quiet, and sitting still, will not contribute much to the rapid remediation of dyslexia. These students need to be active and involved. They need concrete materials that they can see and feel and manipulate and use for associating and relating new learnings. They need materials that are interesting to them. Finding pictures of items that begin with a certain consonant or vowel sound in a Sears, Roebuck or Best catalog, or circling words that begin with a newly learned consonant blend in their own story or experience chart—all are far more interesting than workbooks and dittoed sheets. This is not to say that there is not an occasional need to use such materials, but only to fit certain needs of individual children at certain times.

Our dyslexic students have already been "workbooked" and "dittoed" to death. They need new and different materials with which to work.

The subhead of this section included the words, *classroom and clinic*. This means the regular classroom in which the dyslexic student sits with all students of his class as well as the special room where the dyslexic receives specific remediation on a regular basis by a specially trained person. *Both* teachers should use materials such as those referred to above. The regular classroom teacher will soon find that not only the dyslexic student but the other students in the class as well will become more motivated, will better retain what they learn, and will be able to transfer skills more successfully.

The Cooperation and Understanding of the Parents

I have found that, on the whole, parents are genuinely concerned about their dyslexic child and have been greatly worried about the problems which he has been having in school. They have brought their child to the clinic and are willing to pay the necessary tuition, which can be a real sacrifice to some. The parents are willing to be inconvenienced and to make all kinds of necessary arrangements to get their child to the clinic each day on time and to pick him up, as well as to make the additional trips if more testing and special remediation are required.

A parent rarely goes about the neighborhood bragging that his child has dyslexia, using the condition as a sort of "status symbol." Yet sometimes this is done. And rarely does a parent feel humiliated for having a dyslexic child, believing the condition is something shameful, that it must mean "tainted" blood in the family, or something to that effect. Yet this too sometimes happens.

Such attitudes change when dyslexia is carefully explained to the parents and they understand just what it means for their child to have dyslexia and what can be done for the child—and how important their love and support is at this time.

I have seen tears in the eyes of mothers—and of fathers—at the relief of finding out at last what was wrong with their child and to know that something could be done about the problem. So often, their instinct had told them that there really was something wrong, that their child was not just being lazy or rebellious in school. Often one hears statements such as, "I *knew* there was something really wrong. I just *knew* it in my heart, but the teacher kept telling me that he was smart and could do the work if he just *tried*, but that he's lazy and doesn't want to work."

I shall always remember when a father asked me to step into my office with him. He shut the door and turned to me with tears streaming down his face. He began with, "I know you think that men shouldn't cry [which I don't think,] but I have to tell you that I am so *relieved* now. We have been so worried, so up-tight, so frustrated for so long. We reached the point where everyone in the family was snapping at everybody else. I don't know how to thank you enough for what you've done for our son, whom we love so much."

The dyslexic child has been through so much in his young life that it is crucial that he have the support and encouragement and understanding of his parents. He must know that they are behind him in all his efforts to improve, and that he has their love no matter what has happened in the past or may yet happen; that they will love him in spite of his poor schoolwork, low grades, and occasional outbursts of frustration.

The cooperation and support of parents is also needed by the classroom teacher(s) and by the reading specialist or other special person who is alleviating the dyslexia. Understanding the child's behavior at home, reducing the pressure for high grades, showing an interest in the progress of the child, however small this might be at first, expressing positive feelings about the teachers and what the school is doing for the student—all will help those who are working with your child.

The Cooperation and Understanding of the Classroom Teacher

It is not easy for a teacher to have a dyslexic student in the classroom who needs special work prepared at a level which he can do successfully. Books must be gathered about the specific topics in the curriculum at his lower reading level. Textbook chapters will have to be rewritten at an easier reading level. Directions may have to be repeated. Help must be given with any note-taking, and other adjustments will have to be made in instruction and achievement expectations.

Teachers already work hard for all their students. Planning effective lessons can take hours each week outside of the regular classroom day. While it is customary for secondary school teachers to have at least one period free during the day which can be used for planning lessons, making materials, grading papers, keeping records, and the like, there is never sufficient time, and the teacher often finds that the afternoons, evenings, and weekends must also be used for these purposes. If the teacher is also a coach of some sport, or adviser of a school club, or if there are grade-group or other faculty meetings, the afternoons may not be available either.

Most elementary school teachers have no daily break at all—no reserved time for such planning and teaching preparation. Their afternoons, too, are often filled with school responsibilities other than teaching.

The point is: Teachers are BUSY people. They *have* to care about children and enjoy teaching to work so hard! And when there are special students in the classroom who need additional attention, teachers must work even harder. They do this because they are conscientious, professional persons dedicated to teaching and helping young people. They know the results of their labor can be well worth the effort and time. But they also know that their responsibilities extend to all the students in their class, not just to the dyslexic student.

The classroom teacher needs to work cooperatively with the parents and with the reading specialist who can offer suggestions on how to work with the dyslexic in the regular classroom, and who can help to gather special materials that may be needed. The teacher should not hesitate to ask any questions of the reading specialist, who also serves as a resource person.

Understanding that the dyslexic student is working hard to help himself, that he cannot change the fact that he has dyslexia—and wishes he hadn't— that he needs special attention, and that his condition is extremely frustrating to *him* (as well as the teacher), this understanding will help the child, the parents, and the specialist working with the dyslexic. And it is so very necessary for all those concerned.

The Duration and Frequency of Periods, and Length of Remediation

The amount of time allowed for each period of remediation, the number of times each week the specialist works with the dyslexic student, and the continuation of the remediation until his condition has been alleviated—all will affect the progress of the dyslexic. Much more can be accomplished in hour-long periods than those lasting only thirty minutes. Remediation five times a week will result in faster progress than two or three times a week. It may take a year, or two, or longer to show significant results.

Working with dyslexics two to three hours a day for six weeks in our summer clinic has accomplished notable improvement, but we always advise that this is only a beginning. Parents and students must undertake any program of remediation with patience.

Remediation: One-to-One or Small Group?

The fastest remediation can be achieved on a one-to-one basis; that is, one person working with one child on that particular child's special needs. All the efforts of the specialist are centered upon the child and his needs. The child has no other children to distract him from what he is learning.

This is usually the situation when parents hire trained reading specialists to remediate their dyslexic child on a private basis. There is a financial cost, but parents tend to consider the faster remediation well worth it.

The higher the grade in which a child is placed, the more important reading, spelling, writing, listening, and speaking become. This is due to the heavy vocabulary load in textbooks, the preparation of science and social studies reports, the lecture method of teaching, the need for note-taking, and the additional homework assignments involving reading and writing exercises.

At our clinic we have found that a one-to-two ratio can work well if students are carefully matched according to age, grade, needs—and sex. Two boys or two girls together, not one boy and one girl. We learned the hard way that at any age both girls and boys are very conscious of each other, can be easily embarrassed or become flirtatious, thus detracting from the task at hand. To provide opportunities for social growth and mingling of the sexes, there are times when a teacher will work with small groups or when all the students form one group for a particular purpose.

Most public (and private) schools do not have the resources for remediation on a one-to-one or one-to-two basis. Remediation of those students having problems is usually done in groups of from six to ten or more. In those cases, remediation will occur at a slower rate (less individual attention)—unfortunately for the dyslexic student.

Note for Chapter 13

1. Anita N. Griffiths, *Teaching the Dyslexic Child*. (Novato, Calif.: Academic Therapy, 1978), p. 35.

CHAPTER
14

WHAT CAN PARENTS DO?

Not everything that is faced can be
changed; but nothing can be changed until it
is faced.

—Anon.

The very first thing that you, as parents, must do after an accurate diagnosis is to face the reality of the situation and accept the fact that your child has dyslexia. Admit it to yourselves. Admit it to others. It is not something to hide. Be thankful, in fact, that the dyslexia has been discovered, because now your child can get help for his problems. Now positive steps can be taken. Dyslexia is nothing to be ashamed of—any more than a broken leg or tuberculosis or diabetes. This is no indictment against your performance as parents nor your family genes nor your own intelligence. Dyslexia is a disorder about which something can be done. Your feeling should be one of relief, for you have known that your child has had a problem. Now you know what it is.

The second thing that you must realize is that remediation will take time. There is no magic pill, no instant cure for dyslexia. At the same time, dyslexia should not be used as a "cop-out," nor as a "status symbol." Sometimes one overhears parents and teachers saying, "Johnny can't learn to read or spell; he has dyslexia."

Well, no and yes. Johnny can. And Johnny will.

Your perception of dyslexia and how you handle the situation is critical to your child's success in overcoming his difficulties, for he will sense your feelings and react accordingly—with hope or despair, with faith or doubt, with confidence or uncertainty, with courage or fear. He must know that you love him, that you accept him with his problem, that you do not resent the restrictions that may have been placed upon the family, such as tighter finances if private help must be obtained. Always keep in mind that he loves *you*, and that he really is sorry for any problems which he has caused you at home and at school, and for which he has been carrying guilt feelings for some time.

Again I say there should be a sense of *relief* to find out exactly what has been causing your child to have so many problems in school, to know that he really is not lazy nor being deliberately disobedient. There should be a lessening of worry and tension in the whole family now.

The Home Environment

Show your child that you care about him. Make it evident by your actions that you miss him during the day while he is at school. Give him a big hug when he gets home or when you get home from work. Hold him close for a minute or two—Dad as well as Mom. Ask him about his day—and *listen* to what he tells you. Share some of your day's experiences with him. Draw him into your family discussions. Try to arrange dinner time so that all family members can eat together and share their day, and never let this time degenerate into arguments. Leave the television off at mealtime so that you can give each other your undivided attention.

Show an interest in the papers your child brings home from school. Ask him to tell you about them. Look for the correct things on the papers and comment on them. In other words, commend him for the parts that are well done and let him know that you are aware he is trying very hard at school to do his best. Keep your cool about low grades and papers covered with red ink. Never lose your temper nor ridicule your child about his schoolwork. Remember dyslexics are very sensitive, and the situation will change in time. As he progresses and his work improves, be sure to let him know that you are pleased with the improvement and his hard work. He needs your support and approval very much. Make sure he gets them.

A Quiet Work Place

Parents can help by providing a quiet place where the child can do his work—away from the distractions of the television and movement of the rest of the family. If the apartment or house is small, set aside each school day a certain time for schoolwork to be done by all the children and use the old-fashioned tradition of the kitchen table. At this time, the television and radio should be turned off. Why not pick up a magazine and book to read while the children are working? Sit at the table with the others and read quietly. Your presence will be appreciated and will provide a certain measure of security, for they know you are there if help is needed. Your felt presence will also help keep the children to their task.

Helping With Homework Assignments

I hope that any assignment which your child brings home will be at a level that he can read with ease and understanding, whether books or dittoed work sheets. Sometimes, though, a child with dyslexia will have a teacher who finds it difficult to individualize instruction and prepare work at varying levels. It's "READ OR FAIL" with some teachers, unfortunately. Parents and older children in the family can help the child with dyslexia by using a tape recorder and taping chapters of his textbook on cassettes. The dyslexic can then listen to this taped material as often as he needs to and can stop the cassette at places that he needs to have repeated. He can also listen to the tape as he "reads" along in the book, following the words on the page. This will help him learn new words. Whoever does the taping can later discuss the chapter with the dyslexic. This will help his understanding of the new concepts and will aid in clearing up any misunderstandings which he may have about the material in the book.

If you are thinking, "What! Tape a *whole* book!"—hold it. This is not such an awesome task when you realize that the book may be taped in chapter sections. You only need to stay one or two chapters ahead. The book can be done piecemeal.

Your child will know that all of you are truly interested in helping him when you or his brothers or sisters take the time to help him in this way.

It may be, of course, that your child will be fortunate enough to have a teacher who has already taped the various chapters and you need only to check these out. Still, it would be helpful if you could take the time to listen to the material and discuss it with your child.

A Regular Routine

Children with dyslexia need the security of a framework of routine within which they can function. Try to stick to a regular time for meals and going to bed. Avoid late television for your child, because this interferes with his getting enough sleep, not just because of the late time but because he will be stimulated and for a while will be unable to relax and fall asleep. Your child needs to be rested and alert during the day in order to learn. If he is tired and sleepy he will be more likely to give in to his frustrations—and the tolerance level is always low for a child with dyslexia.

A mother once said to me, "How do you get a child to stop watching TV?" My answer to her was simple: "All TVs come equipped with a button. Just turn it off. After all, *you* are the parent." I did not intend to be either curt or face-tious. I suppose I just wanted her to use her common sense in such matters.

Giving Directions

Your dyslexic child has trouble following oral directions, especially if there are several given at one time. No doubt you have found yourself be-coming exasperated when he has not done what you told him to do. Keep in mind that he is not being deliberately disobedient. He did hear you, but he cannot remember all that you say and he tends to get what he hears all mixed up. He cannot help this. But there are ways you can help him with directions:

1. Keep your directions clear and short; avoid "wordiness."
2. Give only one or two directions at a time.
3. If you need to give more than one or two directions at a given time, write them on paper in list form, as done here.
4. Go over the list with your child.
5. If there are words that give trouble, draw a picture of what is to be done—for example
   "Make your bed."
   "Hang up your clothes."
6. Have your dyslexic draw a line through each direction when it is completed.
7. Post the list in the kitchen, in his bedroom, in the garage, in the tool shed—wherever it is to be used—for easy reference and so as to prevent the list from being misplaced or lost.

Reading Together

In years past it was a common practice for families to read together. Often this consisted of reading the Bible around the kitchen table. Some fam-ilies often read other books together—classics, fairy tales, histories. Read to your child from books of his selection as often as you have time. Share por-tions from your book or magazine that are especially interesting. Encourage him to read silently while you read a book or article of your choice, giving him help as needed with unrecognized words.

Your child will need books that are at a reading level which he can read easily and with enjoyment. There should be no struggling and no frustration. This is sometimes called his "free reading level" or "independent reading level." Your child's teacher will know the level appropriate for him. Do not hesitate to ask the teacher to send home books for this extra reading at home. If you find that he is missing too many words (more than one or two out of a running one hundred words in a passage) and he seems to be struggling and not enjoying the material, or if he refuses to read, return the book to the school and tell the teacher. I should not have to add that these leisure reading books should be about things that are of interest to your child.

Appendix C includes lists of publishers (and their addresses) of books written at lower reading levels for older students who have had problems in learning to read. These books are not babyish and will not embarrass your dyslexic child. Most of the stories and topics should interest your child. When you find out your child's independent reading level from the teacher, you may want to write to some of the publishers and request a catalog from which to order. These books will make good presents for birthdays, Christmas, and just "I think you are great!" gifts.

You may wish to purchase Nancy Larrick's *A Parent's Guide to Children's Reading* [1] which can help you in selecting books to read to your child or for him to read.

What about those monthly children's book clubs? I urge caution here. Often these books are not at the appropriate reading level for your child really to enjoy them. Even children who are "normal" readers will have trouble with some of the books. I have heard parents say, "I don't understand it. That book he's reading came two years ago. He refused to read it then, but now he says it's a good book." Of course, you could read these books *to* your child if they are too hard for him.

It is important that your child see you reading and enjoying books and magazines. Parents serve as models for their children to emulate. Children whose parents sit glued before the "tube" night after night are not going to place a high priority on learning to read.

Shopping Together

Take your child shopping with you. Talk about the prices of foods. Discuss the bargains and how much you may be saving. Compare prices by weight. Take along a small hand calculator. Let him total the prices as you select the items for the week. (But check his entries so you can call his attention to reversed and transposed numerals.) Show your child how to compare prices by weight. Talk about good nutrition and why you buy certain foods even though they may not be the favorites of all in the family. Ask him to take on the job of recording the food needs at home and making up the grocery list for the week—with your help as needed, of course. Writing words will help with his spelling and reading. This will also help to focus his attention on some of his particular difficulties and thus be alert to the occurrence of these errors.

Planning Trips

Trips are usually planned by the parents. Include your dyslexic child (and other children) in the planning. Sit down together with the road map and talk about the trip together. Ask everyone to make a list of what should be taken to the beach, the mountains, the camping trip, to grandmother's, or wherever you plan to go. Then discuss the contents of all the lists and make one master list together. If possible, get extra maps or make copies of your marked map so that each member of the family has one showing the roads to take. If traveling by airplane, try to get the airline's map and use it to discuss the states or countries over which you will be flying, the direction of the route, how fast you will be flying, and how long it will take to reach your destination.

When in the car, call attention to the different signs and billboards. See how many your child can read—always gently giving him help whenever he needs it. Point out special features of letters and shapes of signs and words.

These activities should be looked upon as fun for all, not a chore. Make games of them. And when your child begins to show that he is losing interest in some such activity, discontinue it.

Journal of Important Events

Suggest to your dyslexic child that he keep a record of the family's important events. This does not have to be kept every day, but it should be kept at least weekly. The small books with blank pages available in most bookstores are ideal for this purpose. Tell him that you will help him to spell any words when necessary, but he should try to spell them first. Suggest ideas for entries in the journal. Try to find a daily occurrence that could be recorded. Once a week let him read to the family his record for the week. Parents who have followed this suggestion have told me that the journal is an enjoyable experience for the whole family, and they look forward to the reading each week!

Keeping a Diary of Feelings

Give your child a diary, preferably with a small lock and key. Tell him it is for his eyes only, his privacy will be respected. The diary may be used to write down certain things or incidents that have caused him to have special feelings. He can write what happened from his viewpoint and how it made him feel. The diary should include special things or incidents that made him happy, or excited him, or made him angry, or sad. His dreams and aspirations, his fears and worries can all be written in the diary.

"Get it out and get it down!" should be his motto. Help him to view keeping his diary as a kind of talking to himself. It is amazing how such a diary will help the child with dyslexia to come to terms with himself, to understand why he reacts the way he does sometimes, and in time you will find that he will begin to share some of the things which he has written in this special kind of diary. This sharing should always be voluntary, of course. He must know that you will not invade the privacy of his diary unless he chooses to reveal what he has written.

Helping at Home

A family plays together. A family works together. Chores around the home are the responsibility of all. Encourage your child to help in the kitchen as you cook, with setting the table, working in the yard, or on the car. Foods are cooked in a certain order. Setting the table is done according to a certain form. Chores in the yard and repairs to the car are also done in an order. All these will help your child with his sequencing problems.

When cooking, call attention to the words and pictures on the cans and boxes of food. Let him open them. Ask if he can tell you what sound the word "bean" (or "asparagus" or "rice" or "lettuce") begins with. (Answer: the *b* sound—not *buh*.) He will be associating the concrete items with the abstract phonemes (sounds). Do this when you set the table, or put clothes in the washer, or work in the yard or on the car.

Make all this fun and entertaining. Enjoy these activities yourself! It really *can* be fun. When your child gives you an incorrect answer, just smile and say, for example, "No, fork begins with the *f* sound."

Passing Notes

It does not take long to write a short note to your child telling him that you love him or like something in particular that he has done, or asking him to help you with something. Then in the note ask him to write you an answer. Set up a "family mailbox" in the kitchen or on the porch. Do *not* criticize the spelling errors! Be patient. Just keep writing him notes, and reading and answering the notes from him. You will find that the spelling errors will become less frequent in time.

Slip short, cheery notes in his lunch box, his math book or reader, or in the pocket of his jacket or sweater or pants. Notes like:

— Have a nice day! See you this afternoon.
— This weekend we'll have a picnic in the backyard. What would you like to eat?
— We're having your favorite dish for supper tonight. Yes, it's fried chicken.
— Those were good papers you brought home for us to see. We're proud of your hard work.
— Keep trying! You're doing fine.

And always at the end be sure to write, "Love, Mom (or Dad) or Mom and Dad."

Helpful Games to Play

"My Father Owns a . . . "

Games such as, "My father owns a grocery store [which may be purely imaginary,] and in it he has something that begins with an 'A' or, "My father owns a toy store and in it he has something that begins with an 'A' "—with the correct answer giving an item beginning with the required letter, such as "apple" or "asparagus" or "almonds" (or "air gun" or "airplane" or "anagrams game" if it's a toy store)—can be most worthwhile for the dyslexic child and fun for all. On trips it helps the time pass quickly and keeps everyone in good spirits.

You can vary the categories to keep the games interesting. For example, you might try, "My father owns a . . . ":

drug store	pet shop	cafeteria
book store	zoo	aquarium
circus	farm	ice cream shop
carnival	meat store	used car lot
beach shop	fruit store	furniture store

Games such as these can be played at home, in the back yard, at the pool, on the way to the grocery store or, as mentioned, on trips. How can they help? In several ways: by developing a sense of sequencing and reenforcing knowledge of the alphabet, by using recall, by naming objects and associating these names with the beginning letters, by developing vocabulary, and by using auditory memory.

Let's Pretend

Act out a story commonly known to all family members, or an old familiar fairy tale, or a television show that all have watched together. Here again, memory is being brought to the fore, attention must be paid to the sequencing of events, vocabulary is being developed and used, associations are being made, and feelings and attitudes of characters are being brought out into the open. If your child gets the events out of order, talk about what came first, then next, then next. If he makes other mistakes, discuss these together. For example, point out why a character may have behaved or responded the way he did.

Alphabet Meals

Let one night in each week be a special alphabet letter evening. This is a lot of fun and can present a real challenge at times. Choose the first letter of the alphabet. Together, as a family, try to plan a nutritional meal of foods that begin with that letter. Next week, choose another letter. I recommend that you begin with the letter "A" and proceed in sequence through the alphabet. Each week ask the question, "What meals have we already had?" Answer: "Meals that begin with *A, B, C, D, E,* and next we should think of foods that begin with *F.* Your dyslexic child needs practice with sequencing and reviewing the alphabet whenever he can get it.

Here are some examples of foods for meals for the letters *A* and *B*:

A Foods	*B* Foods
apple cider	banana milkshake
a la king chicken	beefburgers with brown gravy
asparagus, acorn squash,	biscuits and butter
or artichokes	beans, beets, broccoli, or
almond rice	brussels sprouts
avocado or aspic salad	baked potatoes
angel food cake or	butterscotch or Boston
apricot pie	cream pie

This appears to be simple, but you'll discover that remembering a variety of foods beginning with a particular letter is not always easy, especially for some letters. Try to recall the foods at first without anyone referring to a cookbook, though you may have to as a last resort. You may have to use your imagination and improvise a little, which can generate whoops of laughter. For example, for *Y* you may have to resort to "yesterday's left-overs perked up with yeast bread, and yellow cake for dessert." Of course you could come up with "yolk omelettes or yams with ham, and yellow squash." The letter *Z* is a real challenge! You may have to reach as low as "zoo stew with zesty seasoned onions and a zippy dip made of zucchini." Your ingenuity will really be needed for the letter *X*, and you may have to devise such foods as "X-tra long hot dogs or X-citing fruit salad." This is fudging a bit, but what can you do with *X*? After all, it's just a game, and the nonsense makes it even more fun.

One last suggestion for this family game: Be sure to write out the menu on a card or poster so that the menu can be read by all. You want your dyslexic child to *see* these food words as well as *hear* them. He will be getting experience in associating items of food with the beginning letter and sound. He will also be getting experience in trying out new foods and discovering new tastes as well as learning about balanced diets for good health. All this will aid him in developing a store of associations which are being made in a concrete, sensory way and which will probably stay with him permanently.

Let's See!

At any free moment during the day, or on trips by car, whether to the grocery store, school, or next state, play the game of *Let's See!* It is a good deal of fun and does help the dyslexic child. Take turns listing words for things seen along the way. "I see a road and road begins with an *r*" or, "I see a church and church begins with *ch*." The catch is, each time someone "sees" something and says the name and the beginning letter(s) he has to repeat all the words seen before. For example, "I see a horse and horse begins with an *h* . . . road,

church, horse." Since this is just a game that is to be enjoyed by all (while helping the dyslexic child with his recall of words, association of letters with words,
auditory memory, and sequencing), it is permissable to give a little help when
needed. The game stops when everyone bogs down. Then it starts all over
again with one word.

Helping Your Child: Things to Avoid Doing

Avoid Comparisons

I cannot emphasize too strongly the need for you to accept your dyslexic
child as he is and not compare him with any of his brothers and sisters. It does
not help the dyslexic child at all to be told, "Your sister is two years younger
than you and yet she is reading better than you are," or, "Your brother was
reading in a book a year ahead of his grade when he was your age."

A child with dyslexia knows quite well that he has not been living up to
expectations nor achieving at the levels of his brother or sister, whether
younger or older. Please do not take the heart out of him by such compari-
sons. Just believe in him and have faith that he will progress. Give him the support and encouragement that he needs so very much. Let him know that you
understand that he is doing the best he can at the present time.

Watch Those "Put-Downs"

There is a natural amount of kidding and bantering that goes on within
a family, and this is usually healthy for family relations. But there is one kind
that usually takes place between older and younger children that can be harm-
ful. The child with dyslexia is thin-skinned to begin with, very sensitive, and he
does not have a strong, positive self-concept. He harbors certain feelings of in-
adequacy and insecurity, although he may put on an air of not caring that can
fool some people.

Often these put-downs by an older brother (or sister) are only meant to
be funny. The problem is that they don't come across that way; they are taken
seriously by the dyslexic child. A younger child tends to look up to the older
one. The young boy admires his older brother and emulates him. He may
even put him on a pedestal—he can do no wrong in the eyes of the younger
child, what he says is Truth.

So when the older brother comes out with a crack such as, "Hey, stupid,
watch where you're walking!" or, "What a dumbbell!" or, "Hey, birdbrain,
what's the matter with you? *Anyone* knows that word!" the young dyslexic wonders if his older brother really thinks he's dumb and stupid and a birdbrain.
After all, look at all the problems he's having with reading and spelling and
writing and math and everything. Deep inside, the dyslexic has long wondered

if he has inferior intelligence. Put-downs only make him hurt inside, and cause him to feel different from others, and inadequate.

If this particular kind of put-down bantering is going on in your family, have a talk with the older brothers and sisters and explain how words such as those used in the examples above are perceived by the child with dyslexia. Tell them that they must not call him by these words. After all, he has a name, call him by that. Also help them to understand the problems he's having and how very important it is for them to let him know that they really care for him and believe in him. He needs help and encouragement from his brothers and sisters as well as from his parents.

Drug Therapy?

I am not referring here to the use of drugs to "cure" dyslexia, but rather to the possible use of drugs with dyslexic children to help parents and teachers in managing them. This is a highly debatable topic. I am not a physician, and therefore I must be careful not to overstep my professional boundaries of training; however, I can speak from experience with children who have been prescribed drugs for various reasons, and my observations of their behavior, reactions, and achievement in the classroom and clinic.

The usefulness of stimulant therapy has been well validated for the hyperactive group. It has not been for dyslexics. Most reviews of studies indicate that drugs have little or no effect on reading performance.[2] So it is questionable that the use of such drugs provides any help at all for the dyslexic child.

But what about the children who are both dyslexic and hyperactive? The drug may help the child in social situations but will leave untouched the dyslexic elements which still have to be taken care of through remediation. What about students who have both hyperkinesis and dyslexia? In this case there may be some justification for the proper use of stimulant therapy.[3] Only a medical doctor can, of course, make such a decision. I would hope there would be follow-through conferences not only with the parents but also with the child's teachers about the effect of the drug on the child's behavior and performance at home and at school.

Based upon my experience with children with all kinds of problems, I have grave reservations concerning the use of drug therapy. Certainly drugs should be prescribed *only* if they actually help the child—not to appease parents or teachers who want the child to "sit still and be quiet." Parents should never seek drug therapy lightly. The side effects can be serious and may actually detract from the child's attempts to do his work as expected. Sometimes children become snappy and irritable with a short temper fuse, or they may develop nausea and cramps or headaches. They may get the "jitters," and may find it difficult to sleep at night and so come to school tired and sleepy and thus unable to learn in class. Some children lose their appetite and become underweight and malnourished, deprived of necessary vitamins and other nutrients to develop normally.

There is another concern with children who are regularly taking drugs, over and above any dependency that may possibly occur. The "pill-popping" habit may continue with them and could lead to more serious drug-taking. Dyslexics have so many frustrations, ego-cutting experiences, and failures that avenues of escape are sometimes sought—escape from the world of unhappiness to a world of chemical fantasies.

When children who have been taking prescribed drugs for behavior attend our clinic for diagnosis of their academic difficulties, the parents are requested to ask the doctor if the medication can be stopped during the testing and the following remedial lessons. In every case, this request has been granted by the psychiatrist or other medical doctor—who, I might add, is always interested in the consequences.

Without exception, no child has had to return to the medication during his stay with us. True, one or two children have had one or two rough incidents of temper and balkiness, but these passed. An environment of acceptance, faith, caring, and encouragement, with varied, brief, structured lessons built on what the child can do, yet structured upon his needs so that he can achieve and can see his progress, and with opportunities to stretch, move around, get the kinks out before settling down again—all seem to be what the dyslexic needs to get a new direction in his life.

Sometimes teachers confuse learning style with hyperactivity and suggest to parents that drug therapy should be considered. One year when I was teaching third grade, there was a girl, Heidi, in my class. She was rather large for her age, exceptionally intelligent, and very energetic. She had apparently driven her second-grade teacher to distraction, if one can judge by certain comments in the cumulative record. "Hyperactive, won't sit still and stay at her desk, wiggles constantly" were typical observations. This particular second-grade teacher kept her students in their seats copying volumes of work from the chalkboard most of the time. She had suggested to the parents several times that they should consider "giving Heidi a drug to calm her down and make her stay in her seat." Her parents were not convinced that this was the answer to Heidi's problems in school.

I found that Heidi would conscientiously do whatever work was given her if she could quietly get up every now and then and walk over to the window, or get a drink, of water from the fountain, or just stand up and stretch. She did not disturb the other children. She would return to her seat, slip into it quietly, and return to her work. This need for activity was part of her learning style. When allowed the freedom to do these things, she was a very cooperative and successful student in every way.

Heidi's story is related here as an example to parents that they need to ask why a child is behaving in a particular manner in school. They should ask the teacher for specific examples of negative behavior, and then they and the child's teacher should explore possible reasons for this behavior. Children like Heidi need no drug therapy.

It is questionable whether the majority of dyslexics need any drug therapy at all. Perhaps what is more important is for dyslexic students to have understanding, flexible teachers who provide an environment suitable to their learning styles and special needs—including opportunities to move about.

The Parents' Relations With The School

What I suggest here will not be easy for some parents because of unfortunate experiences with school personnel. In some cases the schools have been most conscientious in discovering which students have dyslexia and then providing the remedial care for these children. Others have been negligent in this respect. This negligence is not always the fault of either the teachers or the principal of a particular school, and the parents should realize this. The teachers and principal may wish very much to have a qualified reading specialist in their school who can detect those students who have dyslexia and then work with them to alleviate their condition. The decision may well rest with the "central office" and "higher ups" who may not see the need for the funding or who may place a greater priority on other expenditures—enlarging the football stadium or the parking lot.

If your child has been diagnosed elsewhere as having dyslexia and you have been frustrated in your attempts to get remedial help, do not be too hasty in blaming your child's teacher or his principal. Even though you may ask them why this service is not provided, they may not be in a position to help or to give you satisfactory reasons. It will not help either your child or you if you "bad mouth" the school principal for not having the qualified person to work with your child.

The matter should be pursued with the superintendent of instruction, or the superintendent of special services, if there is one, and then if you receive no satisfaction, do not hesitate to carry the matter to the superintendent of schools. This is the person who can take the necessary steps to provide the funds for specialists in the schools to work with dyslexic children. The lonely principal can only ask for such help and dream. Discuss your feelings with the principal but seek help from those above who determine the priorities for the whole school system.

Teacher Conferences

Never, *never* hesitate to request a conference with your child's teacher if you have any questions or are concerned about the progress of your child. This also applies to the specialist who may be working with your child in support of the classroom teacher. Most teachers are delighted to have parents who are truly concerned about their children, who care about their progress, and who want to help the teacher in any way they can.

If your child's teacher has an unlisted telephone number, as some now have, by all means send a note by your child, or a letter by mail, requesting that the teacher call you, giving a choice of times when you will be home. At this time, set up an appointment and go to the school to talk with the teacher of your dyslexic child rather than discuss the matter on the telephone, because you will want to see samples of your child's work and the results of tests he has taken.

Be prepared for the conference. Make a written list of your questions. During the conference, if you do not understand the teacher's "educational jargon," which we all tend to slip into at times, by all means ask her to explain and give examples. If you have not been trained in education you cannot be expected to be familiar with some of the terms used, no matter how intelligent or educated you may be.

If, for example, you child's teacher says to you during a conference, "He has a lot of trouble with his suffixes. He just can't seem to get his prefixes and suffixes straight," and you are not sure what she is talking about—stop her. Ask the teacher to explain each unknown term so you can understand fully what she is telling you about your child. There is no need to be embarrassed about this. It is no reflection upon your intelligence.

If the teacher does not already have available for your inspection examples of your child's work and test results in support of what she is telling you about his difficulties, be sure to ask for them. They will add to your understanding and perception of the situation.

Keeping Your Cool

In most cases, the parents and school are able to cooperate amiably in helping the dyslexic child. Each understands the other's position and all want to do whatever they can to alleviate the dyslexic's problems—the number one priority.

Unfortunately, this is not always the case. At times parents and school personnel seem to lock horns. This may have happened to you when you sought help for your dyslexic child. You may be disappointed and frustrated because the school cannot, or will not, provide the help your child needs in spite of the federal law for handicapped children, PL 94-142. This may be the result of insufficient funding, the priorities placed on funds, the lack of qualified personnel, or disinterest for one reason or another.

The school may want to place your child in a self-contained special education class with children who have all kinds of handicaps, rather than placing him in a regular classroom with a competent teacher who will work cooperatively with the specialist to whom he should go regularly for special remediation classes. Some parents have found that their child has been placed in a class among mentally retarded students, emotionally disturbed students, students with certain physical and other handicaps. The school may want to place the dyslexic child in a crowded special class where individual attention would be difficult. Or it may want to place him with someone who has not had special training in alleviating dyslexia—which could be disastrous.

Whatever the circumstances, you may find yourself becoming anxious about what is happening to your child, frightened that he may not get the remediation necessary to alleviate his dyslexia, angry that the school personnel do not appear to realize the seriousness of the situation, and frustrated about the whole state of affairs. It would be natural to lose your temper, to want to yell and shout and punch someone in the nose. But you can't. Nothing would be accomplished except a worsening of an already difficult relationship.

So, for the sake of your dyslexic child you must remain cool, calm, and collected. His welfare must always be in your mind. Nor do you want to give the school an excuse for writing you off as an "overanxious, unpredictable, emotionally disturbed, terror," or just another "irate parent." You can accomplish more by a courteous, attentive manner—even though you may be boiling inside. It may be that at a later date you will need to ask that your child be excused from school for remedial lessons on a private basis. This trained person should be able to visit the school and work cooperatively with your child's classroom teacher, helping her to understand the nature of a dyslexic's problems, perhaps suggesting special techniques that will help him, and sharing testing results—hence good relations must be maintained. You may even have other children who attend or will be attending the school, unless you move to another area (which some parents have done to get the necessary help for their dyslexic child).

Following is a letter written by the mother of a visual dyslexic boy to a person in the central office of her school system. She sent a copy to me, knowing that I would be interested in her son's situation at school. He had attended our clinic where the diagnosis of his condition was made. We always send to a child's school the results of testing along with the implications of such findings for the child's achievement in school, and with suggestions to teachers of special ways that will help them work with the student. We have found that most schools are delighted to have children tested and to have suggestions on helping them. Teachers appreciate the helpful ideas and often call to report on the progress of the child. Of course, no teacher is "told how to teach."

The mother has given me permission to share her letter with you. The letter was seven pages long and written by hand in small writing, so some parts have had to be omitted. Nevertheless, the thread of frustration, anguish, and despair with her son's experiences in this particular school system pour through her words. Names have been changed.

Dear Mr. Johnson,

I have two children in advanced classes and one in the gifted at Main School and I know your contribution to this system has made this possible for them to achieve to the best of their ability.

My concern is not for my other three children but for my ten year old in an L.D. [Learning Disabled] Classroom in Grace School . . . My child, Tommy, was placed in an L.D. Class when he seemed to be out in space, as told by his first grade teacher . . . When they placed him in the L.D. system, naturally I became curious when I couldn't find out what his problem was with reading. I felt that surely they would have professionals that would immediately diagnose his problem but I was in for a rude awakening . . . I was told by the school psychologist that my child walked funny, that something was wrong with him as he breathed with his mouth open which was a sign of a mental problem . . . I explained . . . that all my children walked funny as they had crooked legs, that they all breathed through their mouths as they had asthma, allergies, and bronchial problems . . .

[A year later] still not knowing why he was an L.D. student I got in touch with Dr. Anne Marshall Huston at Lynchburg College . . . She did numerous tests and found that he had visual dyslexia. She recommended a private reading teacher and she also was kind enough to send a letter to his teachers telling them the best methods to teach him. Mrs. Albert, his teacher at Grace School, said she didn't appreciate Dr. Huston telling her how to teach and if he had a private reading teacher, she [that teacher] would teach as she [Mrs. Albert] told her to . . . She [Mrs. Albert] had never heard of dyslexia . . . Mrs. Albert's animosity toward me for seeking outside help for my child was met to her satisfaction by taking out her spite on my child. He could do no right. When he finally realized this he did everything he could to stay out of her class. This last year was spent in the office helping the janitor. He became so disturbed and disoriented that now he has a real social problem.

Mrs. Smith agreed to place him in her regular science class, against Mrs. Albert's wishes, after I finally convinced the system that he could function in a classroom setting. There, he has no problems, as Mrs. Smith calls out his tests orally, however I asked that he be placed in other classes and I am informed that he is now a behavior problem so these other teachers don't have to take him. I've asked for help from resource teachers that seem to have extra time when I'm in the school, but they don't have to take L.D. children, they only work with slow children. They prefer I don't

get any outside help in reading as this may confuse my child . . .
John Davis [school psychologist] insists that I put my child on
drugs to shut him up . . . I went to my Dr. W. [who] called Dr. Jackson [Superintendent of Schools] and expressed his concern that
John was using this way out to correct these problems. Dr. W. became very concerned when John suggested I change doctors. We
[parents and Tommy] decided to go to Dr. Lasser [private clinical
psychologist] at $65 an hr. and she also felt that Tommy didn't
need drugs. She and Dr. W. were also nice enough to take their
time and attend our last [school] meeting . . . to prove their point.
We are trying to keep kids off of drugs, not to put them on it.

I wrote a similar letter to Dr. Jackson [Superintendent of
Schools] during the summer and he was very nice to inform me
that he would pay closer attention to the L.D. system and also that
Mrs. Albert would be leaving . . . This year the children . . . have a
concerned teacher, Bob Wilson, but without any help other than
an aide, he can't accomplish miracles. He has a combination of
hearing problems, reading problems, wheelchairs, abused kids,
gifted kids and any kind of kids that regular teachers are not required to take . . . Please get in touch with someone that cares and
get additional help for these teachers so that they can accomplish
more than their checklists and provide adequate education for
each child in these centers. It's spend the money now or destroy
them and their parents and let society pay later.

I apologize for this monologue but hope you will understand
my . . . sincerity in hoping that all of these children will have an
equal opportunity to function.

Sincerely,

Gladys W. Fisher

Private Help For Your Child

If your school has no one trained in working with dyslexics, and if there
is someone in your area who is trained in the diagnosis and remediation of
dyslexia and will work privately with your child on a one-to-one basis, by all
means secure this help. This will add to your financial burden and may represent a sacrifice for the whole family, but in the long run the expense will be
worth it. A professional person who knows exactly what to do, who has the materials necessary for effective remediation, and who will work with your child
alone will be able to alleviate the dyslexia much more quickly than could be
done in school where he is likely to be in a group of eight, ten, or twelve other
students. Even more effective would be for your child to receive the help not
only of this specialist but also of a trained school person who will work with
him several times a week—the two working cooperatively with the classroom

teacher to alleviate his dyslexia. This, of course, is the ideal situation for the dyslexic child, but it is not always possible to obtain.

The time factor is of the utmost importance. As your dyslexic child moves up the grades, his work in textbooks will increase, whether in math or social studies or science or English. The sooner he is helped with his reading and writing and spelling, the better the student and the happier the child, and the more contented you, his parents, will be.

Due Process and What This Means to Parents

Public Law 94-142 (and Section 504 of the 1973 Vocational Rehabilitation Act) has provided certain legal safeguards for parents of handicapped children.[4] Due Process is an example of such legal safeguards.

You have the right to know what the school is planning with regard to the identification, evaluation, and placement of your child. School personnel must consult with you, involve you, and include you in all of it. At the conferences, if you do not understand some of the professional terms used, ask for an explanation. If you wonder about the purpose of certain tests—that is, what information they are seeking—do not hesitate to ask why they are being given to your child. If you do not agree with what is suggested by the school, you may present evidence to contradict the school's recommendations and planned course of action. You also have the right to suggest your own proposals for the education of your child.

Your consent, as parents, is required for the placement of your child in any special education class. In other words, you do not have to agree to this arrangement if you do not believe it is appropriate for your child. Actually, your dyslexic child is likely to do better in a regular classroom—*provided* the teacher understands his special needs and is willing to take him as he is, adapting the instruction, teaching him at his current level of achievement, and modifying performance expectations until his difficulties have been alleviated. Your dyslexic belongs in the regular classroom with a caring and understanding teacher, sensitive to the dyslexic child's anxieties, and one who can be flexible in instruction and the use of materials.

Your dyslexic child also needs on a regular basis the help of the school reading specialist if the specialist is trained in the remediation of dyslexia. This was discussed in the previous section. *Be sure to inquire about this person's specific training in dyslexia.* There are both reading specialists and learning disability teachers in the schools who have not had this training. If the school does not have such a qualified person, then you must seek additional help on a private basis. If your child is excused from school to get this outside help, as is done in some school systems, you will probably be responsible for the transportation. This may be inconvenient for you, but the important thing is to get the necessary help for your child.

In your conferences with the school, try to keep in mind that usually they are sincere people who are earnestly trying to help your child. Their views may differ from yours, and you may strongly disagree with what they recommend. Keep calm and listen to what they have to say. Then present your case in the same manner, courteously and firmly. Parents of dyslexic children have often gone through so much and have had so many frustrations that this is not always easy to do.

The following is a list of rights which some parents may not know they have:

1. You must receive written notice as to the time and date of any hearing.
2. You may have access to any and all records about your child.
3. You have the right to get a separate, independent evaluation of your child (other than that provided by the school).
4. You may decide whether the hearing will be open or closed.
5. Your child may be kept at his present grade placement until all due process hearing appeals have been completed.
6. You may have your attorney with you at any hearing.
7. Your child may be present at the hearing if you wish.
8. You may present any evidence or testimony which you have obtained.
9. You may prevent any information or other evidence from being presented if it was not disclosed at least five days before the hearing.
10. You have the right to challenge any testimony of any person or any evidence presented at the hearing.
11. You may request a verbatim transcript (which is usually an audiotape), and there will be a reasonable charge for this, but I strongly urge that you do this as you may need it for future reference.
12. You may appeal the decision of the members of the hearing panel or the hearing officer—you do not have to buckle under if you disagree strongly.

Family Education Rights and Privacy Act (The Buckley Amendment)

In 1974 Congress passed the Family Education Rights and Privacy Act (FERPA). Parents and their handicapped children now have the right to know what information is in the school cumulative folder and other confidential school records of the child. Do not hesitate to ask to see the "confidential" files, as schools often have two sets of files. Parents may also challenge the comments in the files and correct any errors in the school records. The act also provides one other protection that parents should use: the right of the parents to control the accessibility of the child's school records.

Parents are urged to request to examine these records. This is your child! Ask questions, challenge certain negative comments. Request specific examples of your child's behavior and written observational records to support the negative comments. Does your dyslexic child's records contain comments by teachers such as "lazy, defiant, has to be pushed, is smart but won't do the work, is capable but won't work," and the like? Was he diagnosed as being a dyslexic after these remarks? During? Of course such comments should be stricken from the records of a dyslexic student. Are you aware that your child's academic folder and other school records may follow him throughout his life?

Under the new confidentiality law you have the right to see any psychological assessment of your child. It may be helpful if a psychologist is present to explain the test results and answer any questions you may have.

Boarding Schools for Dyslexic Students

Sometimes I am asked about special boarding schools for dyslexics. The question usually comes about as a result of the parents' dissatisfaction with what the child's school has to offer in the way of remediation of the dyslexia or the locked horns situation previously discussed in this chapter—the parents just want to get their child "out of that school."

Brochures and catalogs are available from these special schools, but the information must be read with caution. The materials cannot always be taken at face value. Remember: this is advertising material to get you interested and to sell the school. The actual program may not be any different from that which the child is getting at his present school, although it is possible that the curriculum may be somewhat more individualized. Naturally any school considered should be visited by the parents and the dyslexic student. In addition to the usual visit with the headmaster and admissions person, you should visit the classrooms while instruction is going on. Listen to the teachers and note how they relate to the students. Observe the students and their reactions in class. Are they interested and motivated? Do they appear prepared for the class and do they participate in the discussion? Are they considerate of their classmates? Stop the students on the grounds and outside of classes and ask them how they are doing in the school, if they are progressing, and so on. Note their attitude toward their teachers and the school as a whole. What individual attention will your child be getting?

These special boarding schools tend to be very expensive. Parents must give careful thought to whether what their child is going to get is really worth the high tuition and probable family financial sacrifice it will entail. You also need to find out if your dyslexic child truly wants to leave home and go off to school. Remember, he has had many unhappy and frustrating experiences, his self-concept is poor, and he tends to feel insecure and inadequate as it is. He must not think that you want "to get rid of him" because he is such a burden and not the kind of son he thinks you would like to have.

I personally believe that the best situation is for the dyslexic child to remain at home and receive the private remedial help on an individual basis, as discussed earlier. You may have to fight hard (but always diplomatically, of course) to get special help at school. Regardless, your child has you to stand behind him, to give him the needed support and encouragement, and the security of your love and acceptance. He would miss you terribly if you sent him away. You would miss him as much.

Notes for Chapter 14

1. Nancy Larrick, *A Parent's Guide to Children's Reading*, 4th ed. (New York: Bantam Books, 1975).
2. Michael E. Thomson, *Developmental Dyslexia: Its Nature, Assessment and Remediation* (London: Edward Arnold, 1984), p. 226.
3. Marcel Kinsbourne et. al., "Questions People Ask About Dyslexia," *The Dyslexic Child* Drake D. Duane and Paula Dozier Rome, eds. (New York: Insight Publishing, 1979), pp. 23–24.
4. Public Law 94-142, Education of the Handicapped Act of 1975. The implementation of Part B dealing with specific learning disabilities was published in the *Federal Register* on December 29, 1977, and went into effect in September 1978.

CHAPTER
15

WHAT CAN TEACHERS DO?

We are all sufferers from our continued
failure to fulfill the educational
obligations of a democracy. We are all the
victims of a school system that has only gone
halfway along the road to realize the promise
of democracy.
—*Mortimer J. Adler*

A s I have stated, the best situation for the dyslexic student is to be in
a regular classroom (the traditional self-contained type) while receiving
regular help from a specialist trained in the remediation of dyslexia
and who cooperates with the classroom teacher to achieve the best environment and instruction for the student to alleviate his dyslexia. This is a form of
"mainstreaming" which some think is a fairly new concept. It is not. Regular
classroom teachers for years have had children with all kinds of handicaps
who have achieved at different levels in their classrooms—beginning with the
teachers in one-room schoolhouses who not only had students of varying
handicaps but also of different ages and in different grades. Teachers have
been dealing with these problems for years and have been successfully educating young people in their charge.

Fads come and go in education. People are prone to jump on bandwagons before research and experience indicate they are good for our children.

The American "open" classroom concept (so different from that in Great Britain), which abolished the traditional self-contained classroom in some schools and actually tore down walls between rooms so that as many as ninety or so young children were in a large area with several teachers, did not achieve the results predicted. Some students who had learned successfully before found that the distraction of so many people in one area, often talking and moving around, interfered with their learning. Teachers could not get to know the individual students as well as in the traditional classroom, where they were with the same group of children all day each day for the entire school year. Teachers and administrators found that tearing down walls did not necessarily create the "open" classroom—the new concept could be as structured and inhibiting as the old. At last educators have come to realize that an "openness" of learning can exist within the self-contained classroom, which can provide a flexibility of planning and instruction and individualizing not available in a situation where there are large numbers of students in one big room.

I have also stated that the "departmentalized" class procedure is difficult for the dyslexic student. Here he has to move from room to room with each subject he is taking, usually with a different teacher. The pressure is on him to complete his work within the class period. The "tyrant" (the clock) is always on the wall watching him, hurrying him, reminding him that time is slipping away.

The departmentalized class procedure has been customary for older students for a long time, and the dyslexic student will have to accept the situation. Ideally, the teachers will understand the dyslexic's problems and will be flexible enough to make certain adaptations in both instruction and expectations of work. But it is unfortunate that the practice has moved to some primary and elementary schools where young children are expected to be miniature adolescents, able to move efficiently to each class and to adjust to a variety of teacher personalities and methods of instruction from hour to hour. Fortunately teachers' voices are being heard—as are those of parents—and there is already a move to modify the departmentalized class procedure in some primary and elementary schools.

Whatever the arrangement within your school at the present time, you and the specialist working with the dyslexic student will be the two most important people in the school for him. As a matter of fact, if you are in a self-contained or "block" departmentalized situation (several subjects taught by one teacher), you will probably spend many more hours with him than will the specialist. You will provide his security within the school. You will, in a sense, be his guardian. If in the past you have not knowingly had the responsibility of a dyslexic in your class the thought may at first appear to be a little frightening, but you can deal with it successfully—and you will find the rewards worth the effort. The experience can be challenging and even exciting. I have known teachers who have become so interested in working with a dyslexic student that they have, on their own, requested his parents to let him stay a little while after school so that they could give more help with his classroom work. I call such dedicated teachers "angels of mercy." Would there were more!

The Classroom Environment

The environment of the classroom must be one in which the dyslexic student feels secure and safe, accepted and *liked* by his teacher and his classmates. You, the teacher, create the environment that exists within your classroom. As the other students observe your relationship with the dyslexic student, the dignity and respect with which you treat him, your friendly attitude and acceptance of him, your willingness to give him special help, your tolerance of certain dyslexic symptoms which he cannot help—such as the spoonerisms or slow responses to questions—they will pick up these traits and will respond to him accordingly.

In Chapter Thirteen certain instructional materials needed to alleviate dyslexia are described. These materials will be exceptionally helpful to anyone working with dyslexic students. You will find that the materials will also help you with the other children in your class who are having academic problems.

As you will discover, your dyslexic student can participate in class discussions. If he does, give yourself a pat on the back, for it means that he feels a part of the class, wants to make a contribution, that he is not afraid to go out on a limb and take a chance. It means that he feels his response will be accepted. He does not have to be afraid of ridicule.

You should know that sometimes a dyslexic student will be "behind" in answering a certain question. You may have already gotten one response from another student and moved on to the next question when the dyslexic student finally raises his hand and gives a response to the former question. This happens because of the "language disconnection" that occurs at times. His mind is still working on and processing the information in answer to the former question. Your reaction to this is very important. Some teachers, not understanding the nature of the dyslexic student, react with impatience or ridicule. If this happens, he is not likely to volunteer to answer a question again. He is more likely to withdraw mentally and emotionally from a situation that is painful to him.

Remember that *he cannot help this behavior*, any more than we can help a sneeze. Accept his answer to the earlier question. You might say, "That's a good answer. It's the right answer to the question, [repeat the question asked earlier]. Both you and [the other student's name] have given good answers and know the information. Now, back to the question I just asked . . . " By replying in this manner you have preserved his self-respect and yet have courteously and kindly indicated that another question has been asked.

You will also find that not all work for the dyslexic student will have to be individualized and specially prepared for him. Besides, there are likely to be others in the class who have similar problems with reading and writing and learning the subject matter, and need the same concepts and skills. These students can form a group according to their particular needs. If you use the unit method of teaching, then the dyslexic student will be able to read books about the subject (written at his reading level), participate in various groups, and contribute as he is able. If you use one textbook for all students in the class, expecting every student to be at the same place on the same page at the same time, then it will be more difficult for you to work with the dyslexic student. If you have one textbook but are willing to be flexible in your instruction, there are several ways to adapt to the needs of the dyslexic student.

Taping Textbook Chapters and Other Assignments

One way of dealing with the dyslexic's inability to read the textbooks for his various subjects is for the classroom teacher (or a volunteer helper who enunciates clearly) to record (tape) the different chapters. This, of course, need not be done all at once. The chapters can be recorded one at a time as long as they are ready when needed. The dyslexic student can then either listen to the tape at school or take the cassette home overnight, in which case he will need a cassette recorder. I have found that in the few cases where students did not have their own cassette recorder, the parents have been quite willing to get one for their dyslexic child.

The dyslexic student can listen to the voice on the tape and look at the words in the book at the same time. Another advantage is that he can stop the tape and replay it any time he gets overwhelmed with information and needs to pick up the thread of thought. He can replay the tape as often as he needs in order to learn the material.

Textbooks are usually adopted for use for a certain number of years. This means that once you have taped the chapters, you need not tape again until a new textbook is chosen by your school system.

You will probably have other students who are unable to read the textbook required for your class. There are media setups containing earphones whereby as many as six or more students can listen to one tape. You will find that other work and special assignments can also be taped and used in this way by the dyslexic student.

Rewriting Material

Another way of dealing with material in books that are too difficult for the dyslexic student to read is for the classroom teacher to rewrite the material so that it can be read comfortably and with understanding by the student. By doing this, the teacher can make sure that the student is acquiring the major concepts in the curriculum for that particular subject. Some teachers rewrite textbook chapters during the summer so as to have them ready before school starts. They do this not only for their dyslexic students but for their other students who cannot read the textbook with ease. Once a chapter is rewritten, as many copies as needed can be reproduced on a copy machine.

Special Subject Matter Books

For whatever subject you may be teaching, books dealing with the content and major concepts are written at lower reading levels. Some teachers request these books for the use of their dyslexic students and other students unable to read the required textbook adequately. The reading specialist in your school will be able to help you in selecting and ordering these books. You will have to make a list, along with the publisher and address and the prices, and submit it to your principal who must approve the funds. When I was a public school teacher and did this, I found my principals always supportive. I sincerely hope that you will be as fortunate.

Listed in Appendix C are some names of publishers and their addresses which may be of help in ordering your books. Your reading specialist will be able to provide additional ones. Appendix D lists some books and materials for different subjects. These are examples that can be used in adapting your instruction. They will be especially helpful in unit teaching.

Films

There is a saying that "one picture is worth a thousand words." This may or may not be so, depending upon the particular picture. There are films that can be obtained free or at a nominal cost (usually from your State Department of Education), rented, or purchased, which can be used in your classroom to present or reenforce certain subject matter. Films can be helpful to the dyslexic student in learning material which he cannot get from his textbook. They can enhance your lessons and provide some variety in your instruction. It helps to use the visual and auditory modalities at the same time, and the classroom discussion following the film will help to organize the information for the students as well as provide you with insights as to which concepts need to be reviewed.

You will want *always* to preview the film before showing it to your students. You may decide that it is not appropriate after all in spite of what the film's write-up says. If you find it appropriate, then you will know how best to introduce the film to your students, what advance information they will need before they view the film. A preview will also enable you to prepare the questions you will want to use in guiding the discussion after the viewing.

While it is true that ordinarily films should be used sparingly for a generation of students already addicted to watching television, and that films do not have the novelty they once did, for the student with dyslexia educational films are one way to learn new material contained in textbooks that he cannot read on his own.

Giving Directions

Remember that dyslexic students have trouble with both oral and written directions. Give prior thought to the directions that you plan to give so that they will be organized, clear, concise, and to the point, with no ambiguity. Give only one or two oral directions at one time, and always reenforce these visually for the student by writing them on the chalkboard or a chart. Do this when giving directions for homework assignments—and make sure the student copies the assignments correctly.

Think about any written directions you plan to include in a lesson or on a test. Are you certain that your dyslexic student can read all the words in the directions so that he understands what is being asked? If not, read the directions to him. Never, never let yourself fall into the practice of telling students to "read the directions and then do the work"—without being sure they can.

Give Tests and Examinations Orally

You will want to consider giving tests and examinations to your dyslexic student orally. This will remove the threat of his having to read the questions. Read the question to him. Let him tell you the answer. Dyslexics often know the answers to questions which they cannot read, for they pick up a great deal of information by "osmosis" in class and often bring much from their previous background to the class. If they have heard taped textbook chapters, read rewritten material, and seen films about a particular subject, they will probably have learned the information asked for in a test.

Dyslexic students have problems with tests and examinations because: (1) they often cannot read all the words in the test questions and are not sure what is being asked; (2) they have trouble writing out the answers; and (3) their writing is slow and laborious, and they are caught in the limits of time.

You may wish to tape the test or examination. You will find that evaluating the answers will probably be more valid, and you can keep the cassette on file if you desire.

Some teachers are critical of this method of giving a test. Perhaps what needs to be considered is this: Is the test being given to determine what information a student knows and how much he has learned about a particular topic, or as a measure of his reading and speed in writing?

Wait-Time

Keep in mind that the dyslexic has trouble with processing information. He needs more time to think, to make sense of what he has seen and heard, and if asked a question in class, to produce the information in a sensible answer. When you ask the dyslexic student a question in class, wait. Do not expect an immediate answer from him. Give him time to think. Wait at least six (or more) seconds for his answer.

Even regular students respond better when there is a wait-time of three to five seconds on the part of the teacher. The length of the answer increases. There are more unsolicited (but correct) answers from students. And there are fewer incorrect answers.[1]

Give your dyslexic student a chance to give you the answer you expect. Give him time to think. Wait, be patient.

Use Multisensory Techniques

The best way to help dyslexics to make associations and relate ideas and to retain information is to take advantage of all the senses and to use concrete materials in instruction as often as possible. This applies to learning new reading and spelling words, studying the geography of a country, doing arithmetic computations—actually, everything in every subject. The dyslexic student needs to hold and feel, to see and hear and touch, to do and act out, to sing and draw—whenever possible. *Both hemispheres of his brain need to be involved in learning.*

One of the most effective sixth-grade teachers whom I have known was a young man who taught in this multisensory, multiexperience manner. He had a typical heterogeneous class—students of varying abilities and differing achievement, with a couple falling in the handicapped classification. What he did with these students in a school year was nigh miraculous. The children turned from "so-so" pupils into excited, eager, curious, knowledgeable students tuned in to learning.

How did he accomplish this? One example will illustrate. The social studies curriculum required a study of the continent of Africa. Of course, the students also had reading, writing, spelling, arithmetic, science, music, and other information to learn.

This young man had insisted on having a self-contained classroom, even at this grade. Otherwise, teaching the way he did and accomplishing so much with his students might not have been possible.

The students pushed back the desks and chairs in the classroom, and on the floor they drew to scale a large map of the continent of Africa. They drew in the countries with the respective capitals and other important cities, and the deserts, mountains, rivers, and seas and oceans. They brought in sand for the deserts, molded the mountains out of paper-maché, and used blue paper for the rivers and neighboring seas and oceans. They calculated the size of the pyramids and made models to scale. (They didn't realize they were learning math when they were doing all this.) They wrote stories about the Africans and shared these by reading some aloud in class and making booklets of them to be read at free times. They acted out excerpts from Shakespeare's *Anthony and Cleopatra* and excerpts from the biblical Book of Exodus. They made their own costumes and prop materials. They learned to sing "Lady of the Nile" and other relevant songs.

Was he teaching his students the necessary subjects in the "curriculum"? More thoroughly than in any other class, and the students enjoyed it so much that they were not aware of the effort they were putting into the process of learning. Their scores on the required standardized achievement tests at the end of the year? Amazing.

A dyslexic student could fit in well in such a class with the flexibility, individualizing, group work, sharing, reenforcement, multisensory approach to learning, and the opportunities for not only mental growth but also social and emotional growth.

Reading Aloud

The Teacher

Read to your students each day. This will not only help the dyslexic student in your class but all your students. It will help them to make the "Language Connection." Whether you are a fourth-grade, seventh-grade, or eleventh-grade teacher, each day read aloud from a story or a selection dealing with your subject. Your students will listen to you reading and learn new vocabulary and concepts as you read, internalize the flow and melody of our language, and develop an understanding of the relationship between a writer and his reader—who in this case is also the speaker—and the listeners who are the students. This reading aloud need only take ten minutes, with an additional few to talk about what has been read, but a great deal is being accomplished in this short time.

The Student

Do not require your dyslexic student to read aloud in front of the class, whether from the textbook or his reader. Dyslexics are very self-conscious about their reading mistakes and feel humiliated and ashamed when this occurs in front of others. Most regular textbooks are too difficult for the dyslexic to read anyhow.

Even the elementary teacher, during a formal reading lesson, should avoid having the dyslexic student read aloud in front of the others. I have already mentioned the ineffectiveness of the Round-Robin method used by some to teach reading.

If your dyslexic *volunteers* to read a story which he has written, or tell how a certain character said something in a story, or repeat a funny joke he has read and enjoyed, this is different. *This* is coming from *him*. He is not being "made" to read aloud from a particular book—and he knows that he can read what he has volunteered to read.

Reading aloud should be required of the dyslexic only for diagnostic purposes, in a one-to-one situation.

Reading Instruction

Even though your dyslexic student is spending time regularly with the specialist who is working specifically on alleviating his dyslexia condition, you have the responsibility to complement his reading instruction in the classroom. The specialist will help you here. As a regular classroom teacher you already know how to find the instructional reading level of your students, the level used to teach reading when using basal readers. Some classroom teachers are more comfortable if the reading specialist reaffirms this level.

It is of the utmost importance that your dyslexic student not be expected to read a book too difficult for him. As in the case of your other students, he should be learning from a reading book that is at his instructional reading level—or slightly lower if he is more self-confident at this level. It is possible that you will have other non-dyslexic students at this same level. If so, you can form a group of those who have the same instructional reading level.

Somehow, in the past, the myth has arisen that the ideal classroom arrangement for teaching the art of reading is to have three groups, even though in a typical classroom there are likely to be more than three levels of reading. In spite of what some appear to believe, there is no Eleventh Commandment that says, "Thou shalt have only three reading groups." To teach reading effectively (and to learn effectively), there should be as many groups as needed by the students in your class. To do so is to assure that you are providing more effective reading instruction, and that you truly will be complementing the work that the specialist is doing with your dyslexic student.

As a classroom teacher, you are familiar with the overall lesson plan of the basal readers. Keep in mind that the dyslexic student will need to be prepared for any new story in the reader by your introducing the new concepts and the new vocabulary in a manner relevant to him by using concrete materials and multisensory techniques. In no way can the dyslexic learn new words if you simply write them on the chalkboard or chart, read them aloud, and have him repeat them to you. He has to tackle new words and become involved with them!

After reading a story, let him act it out. This will help him with any sequencing problems. Correct him gently if he makes mistakes in the sequence. Let him draw pictures of events in sequence and put these up on the chalk tray and talk about them. Let him make dioramas to illustrate scenes—again with your help in rectifying any omissions. Let him (and others in his group) make charts, maps, illustrations of the characters, and the like.

Always stress meaning—the meaning of new words, the meaning of words as they appear in sentences, the meaning of passages, or the main idea of the story as a whole. Remember that meaning is critical to the dyslexic's success in learning.

Computers

The latest bandwagon that educators are hurrying to jump on is using computers in the classroom. Here, again, one must be cautious in giving either blanket approval or disapproval, especially concerning dyslexic students. I have already mentioned the problems dyslexics have when using computers by reason of their reversing letters and numerals, transposing symbols, and confusing similar letters in words or words similar in appearance, and also confusing similar numerals.

I fear that some teachers will want "to plug" the dyslexic child into these machines and let the computer do the work—which it cannot do. If this happens, it is a neglect of responsibility on the part of the teacher. Students have been "plugged" into workbooks, mechanical tachistoscopes and automatic "readers" in the past, none of which has resulted in much progress on the part of the child, and none of which can take the place of a warm, caring, competent human being.

At the present time it appears that advances in the production of the actual computers (called hardware) have shot ahead of the special programs designed for their use (called software). I do not mean to imply that there are not a number of educational programs available which may be compatible with the different brands of computers which schools have purchased. What concerns me is the content of such programs. There is a saying in the computer world, "garbage in, garbage out," sometimes referred to as GIGO. Reading is a *process*—not an accumulation of bits and pieces of skills that together make a whole. The dyslexic student has already had his share of drill and more drill in isolated skills, so much so that he has enough meaningless debris (garbage) floating around in his brain to clog his learning. Computer programs of drill and practice and more drill and practice fall under the category of "garbage in, garbage out," with the possible reenforcement of errors.

Tutorial types of programs should be evaluated carefully by the teacher. Here the student moves from one step to another by answering questions. One must ask if what is being stressed is really what the student needs. Is the information in each step needed? Or is it more "garbage in, garbage out?" Are there other ways of teaching this information that would be more meaningful and effective?

There are still other programs that contain questionable material. Could anyone trained in education and the nurture of children possibly have designed the program that responds to a mistake by a student with "Wrong answer, dummy!"? Or the one that gives an ugly, mocking, "raspberry" sound when the student makes an error? Students with dyslexia already have a low enough self-concept, and they secretly worry about being really "dumb." They are very sensitive to criticism, especially the put-down type. Such responses, even if made by a machine, only serve to reenforce the dyslexic's negative ideas about himself and to increase his anxiety in learning.

To be able to transfer any new skills and concepts to reading and writing is *essential*. Some teachers have trouble getting their students to transfer and apply new learnings in reading and writing language because they have taught these in isolation to their students. In the same way, I am concerned about the transfer of skills learned from the computer to the actual tasks of reading and writing.

As for the word processor, it may be beneficial in writing papers and its spelling program may catch misspelled words. Still, the dyslexic student will have certain problems, already mentioned.

Careful thought should be given to whether and how computers can help the dyslexic student, and whether the expense is justifiable. Perhaps other means would be more effective given the expense involved—as, for instance, the employment of a full-time reading specialist.

The Reading Specialist in Your School

The reading specialist is able to suggest special activities in the classroom to reenforce what is being done with the dyslexic student in the reading clinic. The specialist can also help in acquiring various materials that you may need and in selecting and ordering other special materials and books suited to your dyslexic student.

The Teacher's Aide/The Volunteer

If you have a teacher's aide or a volunteer mother or other helper, be sure always to give careful instructions as to what they should do—and how they should do it. Keep in mind that their job is not to "teach"—that is your job—but to help you with your dyslexic student while you are working with the other students in your classroom. They can read a story or chapter of a textbook to him, *review* certain skills and new words previously taught by you, help with his spelling, and use the kinesthetic technique for teaching new reading and spelling words. (See Appendix E for an effective kinesthetic approach.)

Do *not* have these helpers simply sit and flash isolated words on cards to the dyslexic student. This is a meaningless drill and can be a frustrating and useless experience for a child with dyslexia. Instead, have them use sentence strips in which the sentence contains the word, which is underlined. (The student should be able to read the sentence, of course.) The word could also be written on another strip piece, and the child could match that word with the same word in the sentence, and then make up his own sentence using the word. The sentence strip could be placed at the top of the pocket chart and the helper could then proceed with another sentence strip. Each time, though, the dyslexic student should read the preceding sentences before moving to another one.

Public Law 94-142 (Education of the Handicapped Act)

In 1975 Congress passed Public Law 94-142 (Federal Register, 1977) which requires the states to provide educational programs for all handicapped children between the ages of three and twenty-one. The right to "free, appropriate public education" for handicapped children, geared to their particular needs, has been mandated for, but not necessarily received by, all handicapped children.

The term *handicapped children* is broad and includes those who are deaf, hard of hearing, mentally retarded, orthopedically impaired, severely emotionally disturbed, speech impaired, visually handicapped, and learning disabled. Learning disability is defined in the regulations for Public Law 94-142 as:

> A disorder in one or more of the basic psychological processes involved in understanding or in using language, spoken or written, which may manifest itself in imperfect ability to listen, think, speak, read, write, spell, or to do mathematical calculations. The term includes such conditions as perceptual handicaps, brain injury, minimal brain dysfunction, dyslexia, and developmental aphasia. The term does not include children who have learning problems which are primarily the result of visual, hearing, or motor handicaps, or mental retardation, or of environmental, cultural or economic disadvantage.[2]

When this law went into effect in September 1978, funds were provided for the states and localities to help in the education of handicapped children. Unfortunately, many superintendents of school systems and directors of instruction and special services were and still are confused as to what services are reimbursable under the law.[3] Consequently, some students who have serious reading and spelling problems are not getting the help they need.

Dyslexia was specifically named in the definition of learning disability in the mandate by the federal government. Nevertheless, in a number of schools the dyslexic student is not getting the kind of help that he needs. There are several possible explanations for this. Some teacher training institutions have not adequately prepared their reading specialists and learning disability teachers in the diagnosis and remediation of dyslexia. In some institutions there are those who deny that dyslexia exists and therefore their graduates leave the college or university ignorant and insensitive to the problems of the dyslexic student. In some public school systems there are insufficient reading specialists and learning disability teachers to take care of the number of students in need. There are few in-service programs dealing with dyslexia to help the public school classroom teacher deal with students who have this disability.

The Age Limits of PL 94-142

The range of ages, from three to twenty-one, has implications for the schools. More and more pressure for early identification of problems is being brought to bear upon school personnel. Certainly we want to identify children with vision or hearing defects, the orthopedically impaired, the emotionally disturbed children, and those with severe speech impediments and brain damage.

But where determining "mentally retarded" can be tricky at the early age of three, and identifying certain speech problems can be precarious, detecting dyslexia at the age of three is ludicrous! The reasons have been explained in Chapter Six dealing with the early identification of dyslexia—before the age of eight—and there is no need for repetition here.

The upper limit of twenty-one years of age means that our high school dyslexic student can remain in school longer to continue receiving special services of remediation. If the young person is able and wants to remain in school—does not have to work—then this is to be desired, as he needs all the help he can get for as long as he can get it. But most young persons, especially those who have had difficulties and frustrations along the way, are anxious to get out of school and on with their lives. I doubt that many dyslexics will continue to stay in school—too many, as it is, drop out of school as soon as they reach the legal age.

The Classroom Teacher's Rights Under PL 94-142

Classroom teachers may have the notion that Public Law 94-142 provides rights only for handicapped students and their parents, and perhaps for the special education professional.[4] This is not the case. You, too, have the following rights:

1. To have a student adequately diagnosed,
2. To participate in the program planning process, especially if a student is "mainstreamed" into your classroom,
3. To work with the education specialist who is alleviating the student's dyslexia,
4. To have adequate resources for your instruction of the dyslexic student,
5. To receive the assistance of parents in complementing the school program at home.

Sometimes regular classroom teachers believe they are considered less important, even less intelligent, than the reading or special education specialist, or the school psychologist, or other special personnel in the school. This may be so although they too have a master's degree from an eminent school of education. The feeling may be due to the fact that often the classroom teachers are not included in some conferences concerning a child, or perhaps their specific recommendations are ignored. They become hesitant about taking the initiative with a child, and reticent about making suggestions which they believe appropriate—standing up for what they know is right. Like the dyslexic student, these teachers begin to lose their self-confidence, and they become sensitive and somewhat defensive. *Do not let this happen to you!* Recall that I began this chapter by saying that you are important to the dyslexic child: "You will provide his security within the school. You will, in a sense, be his guardian." Remember these words and draw courage from them. The dyslexic child in your classroom needs you. Do not let him down.

Individual Educational Program

Public Law 94-142 requires that an individual educational program (IEP) be prepared in detail for each child. Annual overall goals must be set with a list of short-term objectives to serve as steps in achieving each annual goal. Special instructional materials used for each task must be listed along with the criteria for success, and tests and other evaluation procedures to determine if the objectives are being met—if the student is learning what he is supposed to be learning as planned.

The regular classroom teacher may or may not participate in the IEP, depending upon the policy of the particular school.

The advantages often cited for an IEP are:

1. The teacher and other personnel must focus upon the child himself.
2. Individual strengths and weaknesses of the child become known.
3. Progress of the child is noted.
4. The IEP says, "This is where we're going, how we're to get there, and how we will know when we've arrived." [5]
5. Since the parents' approval is required, they are more likely to feel as though they have been involved in the process.

IEP's are criticized for these reasons:

1. IEP's require the spelling out of detailed, specific behavioral objectives which permit only a very narrow definition of both curriculum and competence. [6]
2. In this behavioral approach, various skills are broken down into fragmented pieces, and our dyslexic students already have too many bits and pieces of garbage floating around in their heads.

3. The isolated approach to reading prevents students from un-derstanding what reading is all about. Learning skills becomes the end rather than the means to successful reading. Many of our dyslexics have already begun to internalize this erroneous concept of the reading process.

4. Success criteria of 80 percent accuracy on tasks (or 85 percent or 90 percent or 75 percent) still leave gaps in knowledge and can contribute to additional problems with skills at a higher level. (For example, not knowing the consonant "l" can affect the learning of the "l" blends [*bl,cl, fl* . . .].)

5. Preparing the IEP and short term daily (or weekly) objectives in a professional manner is extremely time-consuming and re-duces the time that could be spent in planning motivating les-sons and making creative materials to achieve more effectively the objectives.

6. While the IEP is supposed to stress individualization, in the sec-tion on procedures, instructional methods, media/materials, and evaluation procedures, lists such as this are found:
"Hayes ditto worksheet"
"Workbook, page 20"
"Workbook, page 21"
"Workbook, page 22"
"Commercial and teacher worksheets"
"Blend ditto worksheet"
"Digraph ditto worksheet"
"Commercial and teacher worksheets"
"Completed worksheet"
. . . and so on . . . and on . . .

7. IEPs too often fail to emphasize the sustained silent reading needed for the transfer and application of skills and new words learned, the creating of experience charts and word banks, and creative writing by students. These activities are all aimed at "meaning" and could certainly be used with IEPs.

To return for a moment to the listed advantages of the IEP, note should be made that conscientious teachers have always focused upon the child as an individual with individual strengths and needs. For years teachers have kept progress charts of various kinds to indicate how well a student is achieving. In order to be effective, all teachers must plan and set objectives—and work hard to meet the overall goals set for students. The only thing new about the IEP is, perhaps, that a separate program must be written for each child.

Programs to Avoid

There are certain commercial programs and kits that have been reputedly good for working with dyslexic students. As we have learned more about the diagnosis and alleviation of dyslexia, we have found that certain programs and approaches are suitable—but others are not. Some to avoid are those that:

1. Do not stress meaning and understanding on the part of students. (This is critical to a dyslexic's success in acquiring new concepts, vocabulary, and skills.)
2. Emphasize the teaching of the phonic elements in isolation. (The rationale for this has already been presented in detail.)
3. Use an orthography other than our traditional alphabet, including color coding of words or sounds or a restructured alphabet to represent the forty-four sounds in our language, or special pictures to represent the sounds of the alphabet or words. (The dyslexic has enough difficulty mastering his own alphabet: the visual dyslexic, with difficulty in revisualization that causes unstable letter formations and incomplete recall of details in pictures; and the auditory dyslexic, with processing the sounds represented by the letters of our alphabet. Moreover, our books are written in traditional orthography and these must be used to transfer the skills learned.)
4. Stress any kind of speed reading, tachistoscope flashing, controlled reading, or fast-paced verbal responses required. (The dyslexic needs *time* to process information. Any pressure for speed and quantity can cause him undue stress.)
5. Require a dyslexic to proceed through workbook pages on his own in a programmed manner, or unsupervised work in workbooks. (The dyslexic has special needs requiring attention. Any program where students go through a workbook working all the pages one after the other is not meeting the individual needs of a student. This "canned" approach will not help the dyslexic who needs guidance and attention to specific difficulties.)
6. Are highly structured regarding what the teacher is to say and do as well as what the child is to say in response. (The dyslexic student needs flexibility of instruction, creativity on the part of the teacher, and individualization based on specific needs.)
7. Permit an undue amount of noise, such as the students' "shouting out" the answers all at once. (The dyslexic student tends to be sensitive to noise and movement, and these will distract him and cause confusion.)

8. Attempt to remediate dyslexia by having the student creep, crawl, balance on beams, jump on trampolines, and the like. (These may be fun for the dyslexic student and perhaps help his coordination, but they will not help his dyslexia condition.)

9. Require spelling lists where the words must be memorized in rote fashion. (Dyslexics need to use the words, associate them with things and experiences in his background, and write the words.)

10. Rely heavily on drills of words and skills in isolation. (The dyslexic needs to use words and skills in context where they will have meaning and be better retained.)

11. Do not use multisensory techniques for learning new concepts, vocabulary, and skills. (The dyslexic student needs to say and hear and see and touch, drawing on his senses.)

12. Ignore the use of concrete manipulative materials. (Again, the dyslexic needs to see and feel; he also needs to smell and hold and manipulate materials representing new concepts. This enables him to make associations, gives him mnemonic cues he can draw on when needed, and makes learning come alive for him.)

13. Emphasize one particular word recognition strategy. (The dyslexic student needs to learn a variety of strategies to help him, for some work better than others, depending on the situation.)

14. Use optical devices and exercises to remediate dyslexia.[7]

15. Use chemicals and vitamins reputed to "cure" dyslexia.

16. Use ridicule or put-down comments when the student makes an error or is confused.

Communicating with Parents

I suggest that you have a conference with the parents of your dyslexic student fairly soon after the beginning of school and that it include the reading specialist or other specialist working with the student. By doing this the parents will see that the two of you are working cooperatively to create the best learning environment and instruction for their child. Later, you may wish to meet with them in your classroom to discuss special things that you may be doing with him and the class as a whole.

Sometimes parents come in with what may appear to be a chip on their shoulder. Try to understand that this is the result of what may be years of frustration and anxiety in trying to get help for their child, to get him placed with a classroom teacher who understands his particular problems. Some parents feel truly battered. Some have been shunted and pushed aside or ignored or ridiculed in their search for help.

Accept the parents as you accept the student with dyslexia: with interest and caring and understanding and faith. Let the parents talk out their problems, explain what has happened in the past, what they hope will happen—and then it will be done. *Listen attentively* to what they have to say. You may be astounded at what information they reveal. Let them know that you are pleased to have their child and will work very hard to help him. This is what parents need to hear.

For conferences with parents, be sure to have samples of the student's work and the results of tests and other papers to show the parents and substantiate the information you are giving them. Keep samples for yourself so that later in the year you and the parents can compare the student's work at various times and see the progress he is making.

Telephone the parents occasionally or send home a short note telling them about something that the dyslexic student has done especially well. This will make the student and his parents happy, and it will show them that you do care and are interested in his progress.

There will be times when you are discouraged. When this happens try to remember that in any child's progress, especially a dyslexic's, there are plateaus and peaks, troughs and crests, crawls and leaps in learning. Have faith in the dyslexic. Trust him. And trust yourself as his teacher.

When report time comes around you may wish to invite the dyslexic's parents in to discuss his marks. Or you may wish to write a special note to accompany the report card. In either case you should begin with the student's strengths and taper off with what he still needs to work on.

When I taught in elementary school I used to write such notes with the report card of every child in my class. I found that this contributed a great deal to good parent relations, and years later when I happened to run into the parents, they would make a point of expressing their appreciation. This takes time—and a thorough knowledge of the student's strengths and weaknesses—but it is well worth the effort.

Most of all, you will find that parents want to know that their child is happy in school, happy with you, and happy with his classmates. They want to know that he is learning and making progress. They realize that because of his special problems you must work harder and longer. While they may not say so, they are grateful to you. Remember that always and resolve that you will never let them down—nor your student with dyslexia—nor yourself as a professional, dedicated teacher. Remember to keep your feet on the ground and use your common sense when working with the dyslexic student—and both of you will learn together.

* * * *

To have striven, to have made an effort,
to have been true to certain ideals—this
alone is worth the struggle.
                                    —*Sir William Osler*

Notes for Chapter 15

1. Mary Budd Rowe, "Wait-Time and Rewards as Instructional Variables, Their Influence on Language, Logic, and Fate Control: Part One—Wait-Time," *Journal of Research in Science Teaching* Vol. 2 (1974), pp. 81, 89–93.
2. Public Law 94-142, Education of the Handicapped Act of 1975. The implementation of Part B dealing with specific learning disabilities was published in the *Federal Register* on December 29, 1977, and went into effect in September 1978, 121a.5 [9].
3. Leslie Burg and Maurice Kaufman, "Laws about special education: Their impact on the use of reading specialists," *The Reading Teacher* Vol. 34, No. 2 (November 1980), p. 189.
4. "The Teacher's Rights in PL94-142," editor's interview with Attorney Reed Martin in *Journal of Reading Disabilities* Vol. 11 (June/July 1978), p. 332.
5. George Kaluger and Clifford J. Kolson, *Reading and Learning Disabilities*, 2nd ed. (Columbus, Ohio: Charles E. Merrill, 1978), p. 215.
6. Lenore H. Ringler and Carol K. Weber, *A Language-Thinking Approach to Reading, Diagnosis and Teaching* (New York: Harcourt, Brace, Jovanovich, 1984), p. 358.
7. *The Role of the Ophthalmologist in Dyslexia*, Report of International Seminar (Melbourne, Florida: Institute for Development of Educational Activities, 1969), p. 10.

APPENDICES

APPENDIX

ERRORS CAUSED BY
INCORRECT PHONICS INSTRUCTION

The following are examples of errors made by nondyslexic students on a diagnostic test given to determine how the phonic elements had been taught to them. The key word confusions are quite logical when one considers how the sounds were taught. Here we have a glimpse of how their minds have used incorrect information to arrive at incorrect key words—words *not* beginning with the blends. Such errors are similar to those of the dyslexic and could result in a misdiagnosis if the examiner is not aware of how the child was taught phonics. If a dyslexic student is taught in this nonsensical manner, his problems will be compounded.

The students said that the—	*And gave one of these words as a key word:*
sound of *br* is "bur"	burn, Bert, Burrhead Jones
sound of *cr* is "cur"	curve, curt, curtsey
sound of *dr* is "dur"	derby, dirt, dirty
sound of *pr* is "pur"	purr, purple, person, purgatory
sound of *tr* is "tur"	turtle, termite, term
sound of *fl* is "ful"	full, Fulton, fullgrown
sound of *sk* is "suhkuh"	sucker, suckle
sound of *sp* is "suhpuh"	supper, superb, support
sound of *cl* is "kul"	color, culprit, cool
sound of *sn* is "sssss (a hiss sound) nnnnnnnn "	sun, sin, soon

APPENDIX
B

TWIN STUDIES

Knud Hermann. *Reading Disability, A Medical Study of World-Blindness and Related Handicaps* (Springfield, Ill.: Charles Thomas, 1959)

Hermann pooled the findings of three studies concerning twins: In one study, Hallgren (1950) used six sets of twins of which three were identical twins and three nonidentical pairs. Norrie (1954) used twenty-eight sets, of which seven were identical and twenty-one were nonidentical. Norrie had also completed another study, unpublished at that time, where she studied eleven sets of twins, of which two pairs were identical and nine were nonidentical.

Of the total forty-five pairs of twins studied, all of the identical twins were concordant. Twenty-seven pairs of the nonidentical twins were concordant (33%). Hermann concluded that "since all the uniovular twins showed concordance, it is evident that heredity is the only decisive factor." (p.87)

Edith Zerbin-Rubin, "Congenital Word-Blindness," *Bulletin of the Orton Society,* 17 (1967), p.50.

Zerbin-Rubin summarized nine studies on twins: Hallgren (1950), Norrie (1954), Brander (1935), Ley and Tordeur (1936), Jenkins, Brown, and Elmendorf (1937), Schiller (1937), vonHarmack (1948), Weinschenck (1962), and Spiel (1953). Of Norrie's thirty-nine sets of twins, all nine identical sets were concordant, with only ten of the thirty nonidentical sets concordant. Of Hallgren's six sets, all three identical twins were concordant, with only one of the three nonidentical pairs being concordant. Single case studies of concordant identical sets of twins were reported by Brander; Ley and Tordeur; Jenkins, Brown, and Elmendorf; Schiller, and vonHarnack. One concordant nonidentical (boy-girl) pair was reported by Weinschenck. Two concordant sets of unknown zygocity were reported by Speil and Weinschenck.

In summary, all seventeen identical twins were concordant, twelve of the thirty-four nonidentical twins were concordant, and two concordant sets of unknown zygocity were reported.

*　　*　　*

Note: While these two summaries of twin studies are often referred to in articles and books on dyslexia, no mention has been made that there may be some overlapping of the results. It would appear that Hallgren's sets of twins are the same for both studies. And are Hermann's seven identical and twenty-one nonidentical sets from Norrie a part of the larger number of twin pairs used in Zerbin-Rubin's summary?

APPENDIX
C

LIST OF PUBLISHERS
AND THEIR ADDRESSES

In this Appendix are given the names and addresses of some publishers who distribute books and other materials which are suitable for working with the dyslexic. Since the names of some publishing companies change; others may go out of business, and addresses change from time to time, you will want to check any in which you may be interested. This can usually be done at your local library. Ask for *Books in Print* which is published each year.

Addison Wesley Publishing Company, 2725 Sand Hill Road, Menlo Park, CA 94025.

Ann Arbor Publishers, Inc. 616 Church Street, Box 1446, Ann Arbor, MI 48104.

Barnell Loft, 958 Church Street, Baldwin, NY 11510

Benefic Press, 10300 W. Roosevelt Road, Westchester, IL 60153

Bowmar/Noble Publishers, Inc. 4563 Colorado Boulevard, Los Angeles, CA 90039

Doubleday & Company, Inc. 501 Franklin Avenue, Garden City, NY 11530

Educational Teaching Aids, A. Diagger & Company, 159 West Kinzie Street, Chicago, IL 60610

Fearon-Pitman Publishers, Inc., 19 Davis Drive, Belmont, CA 94002

Follett Publishing Company, 1010 West Washington Boulevard, Chicago, IL 60607

Garrard Publishing Company, 1607 North Market Street, P.O. Box A, Champaign, IL 61820

Globe Book Company, 50 W. 23rd Street, New York, NY 10010

Janus Book Publishers, 2501 Industrial Parkway, West, Dept. A.M., Hayward, CA 94545

Milton Bradley Company, 74 Park Street, Springfield, MA 01101

Modern Curriculum Press, 13900 Prospect Road, Cleveland, OH 44136

Pendulum Press, Inc., Department C., Box 509, West Haven, CT 06516

Prentice-Hall, Inc., Englewood Cliffs, NJ 07632

Quercus Corporation, 2768 Pineridge Road, Castro Valley, CA 94546

Random House, Inc. 201400 Haln Road, Westminster, MD 21157

Reader's Digest Services, Educational Division, Pleasantville, NY 10570 (Random House handles some of their materials.)

Scholastic, Inc., 2931 E. McCarty St., P.O. Box 7501, Jefferson City, MO 65102

Steck-Vaughn Company, P.O. Box 2028, Austin, TX 78768

Webster (Division of McGraw-Hill Book Company), 1221 Avenue of the Americas, New York, NY 10020

APPENDIX
D

MATERIALS TO HELP
WITH SPECIAL SUBJECTS

Reading Level
(Grade Equivalent)
SCIENCE:

1	*Science for You: You Can See*
2	*You Can Do*
3	*You Can Learn*
4	*You Can Explore*
5	*You Can Discover*
6	*You Can Experience*
2.3	*Wonders of Science: The Human Body, Water Life, The Earth and Beyond, Land Animals, Matter, Motion, and Machines, Plant Life.*
	(Steck-Vaughn Company)

1	*Science Work: Science is Looking*
2	*Science is Measuring*
3	*Science is Comparing*
4	*Science is Inquiring*
5	*Science is Experimenting*
6	*Science is Predicting*

Reading Level
(Grade Equivalent)

| 3–4 | *Insights Into Science* (Interest Level: Students in grades 4–6) |

3–4   *Insights Into Science* (Interest Level: Students
       in grades 4–6)
3–4   *Experience in Science* (Pathways Text) (Interest Level:
       Students in grades 4–6)
       (Modern Curriculum Press)

2.2   *Earth Science*
2.3   *Physical Science*
2.4   *Environmental Science*
2.4   *Human Biology* (also has accompanying lab book)
2.5   *Biology of Plants and Animals* (also has accompanying
       lab book)
       (Quercus Corporation)

5–6   *Pathways in Science*, Revised Edition (geared for junior
       high level students and above)
       Life Science
       Earth Science
       Chemistry
       Physics
       (Globe Book Company)

7–9   *Ideas and Investigations in Science* (geared for junior
       high level students and above)
       Life Science
       Earth Science
       Physical Science
       (Prentice-Hall Educational Book Division)

3–6   *Science Readers* (Interest level: students in grades 3–9)
       (Reader's Digest Services)

Reading Level
(Grade Equivalent)

2.5   *Life Science in Action: Human Systems*
                              Animals
                              Green Plants
                              The Five Senses
2.5   *Earth Science in Action: Earth Resources*
                              Changing Earth
                              Weather
                              The Solar System
2.5   *Physical Science in Action: Energy*
                              Electricity
                              Machines
                              Sound
(Janus Book Publishers)

---

700 Science Experiments for Everyone (Doubleday and Company)

SOCIAL STUDIES
(HISTORY/GEOGRAPHY/GOVERNMENT)

3   *Georgraphy Skills Series: Lands at Home*
4   *Regions of the World*
5   *The American Continents*
6   *Continents Overseas*
       (Interest Level: students in grades 7–8–9–10)
7   *World Geography*
8   *American Adventures* (Interest Level: students in
       grades 7–8–9)

4   *Our Country Today*
5   *Our Country's History*
6   *Our World Today*
5–6   *Our U.S.A., Part 1*
5–6   *Our U.S.A., Part 2*
7–8   *Our Nation's Story, Part 1*
7–8   *Our Nation's Story, Part 2*

Reading Level
(Grade Equivalent)

JHS	*Our Democracy,* 2nd edition (In addition to the above, some state histories may be obtained from Steck-Vaughn Company. These include Alabama, Arkansas, California, Florida, Georgia, Kentucky, Louisiana, Mississippi, Missouri, New York, Tennessee, Texas, and Virginia. Since the reading levels vary, you will need to send for Steck-Vaughn's catalog.)
2.5	*It's Our Government, Congress, the President, and the Courts*
2.5	*Government at Work, from City Hall to State Capitol*
2.5	*Electing the President*
2.8	*Stamp and Story Histories: Highlights of American History*
2.8	*Famous Americans* (Janus Book Publishers)

(Comic book format)

The Basic Illustrated History of America Series
The New World 1500–1700
The Fight for Freedom 1750–1783
The United States Emerges 1783–1800
Problems of the New Nation 1800–1830
Americans Move Westward 1800–1850
Before the Civil War 1830–1860
The Civil War 1850–1876
The Industrial Era 1865–1915
America Becomes A World Power 1890–1920
The Roaring Twenties and the Great Depression 1920—1940
World War II 1940–1945
America Today 1945–1981
(Pendulum Press, Inc. Note: Cassettes and filmstrips are available for the above.)

Reading Level
(Grade Equivalent)

K–3   *Map Skills 1* (RC 01343); Includes basic map concepts, map symbols and legends, map directions, map distance and scale; also includes four sound filmstrips with cassettes.

4–6   *Map Skills 2* (RC 01344); Includes What Is a Map?, Travel Maps, Social Purpose Maps, Political Maps; also includes four sound filmstrips with cassettes.

K–3   *Globe Skills 1* (RC 01345); Includes What Is a Globe?, What Does a Globe Do?, Where Do We Live?, How Do We Get Night and Day?; also includes four sound filmstrips with cassettes.

4–6   *Globe Skills 2* (RC 01346); Includes Hemispheres and Parallels; Latitude and Longitude; Yesterday, Today, Tomorrow; The Four Seasons; also includes four sound filmstrips with cassettes.

1–6   *Success With Maps* (Books A–F)

1–6   *Map Skills* (Books 1–6)
          (Scholastic, Inc.)

---

4   *American Democracy Series:*
          America the Beautiful
          Electing Our Presidents
          The FBI
          The Making of the United States
          The Office of the President
          The Statute of Liberty Comes to America
          Story of the Boy Scouts
          The Story of the United States Flag
          The Supreme Court in America's Story

4   *Living in Today's World Series:*
          Canada, Giant Nation of the North
          Ethiopia, Mountain Kingdom
          Iran, Crossroads of Caravans

Reading Level
(Grade Equivalent)

The People's Republic of China,
Red Star of the East
The Soviet Union, Land of Many Peoples
(Garrard Publishing Company)

2.5–4.0   MATH

Math in Action Series:
Math Language
Understanding Word Problems
Solving Word Problems
Estimation
Using a Calculator
(Janus Book Publishers)

4–6   *Tables, Charts, and Graphs* (Books A–C)
3–8   *Problem Solving in Math* (Books 3–8)
          (Scholastic, Inc.)

2–4   *Math-A-Riddle I*
3–5   *Math-A-Riddle II*
1–5   *Math-A-Dot* (Books 1–5)
          (Fearon-Pitman Publishers)

3–8   *Practicing Problem Solving* (Books 3–8)
          (Random House)

Reading Level
(Grade Equivalent)

HEALTH

1–8	*Choosing Good Health Series* (Books 1–8)
2.3	*Health and You* (two books: Book 1 and Book 2, with interest levels of 5–10 grades)
2	*Steck-Vaughn Health Series: Your Growth*
3	*Growing and Changing*
4	*Your Healthy Body*
5	*Your Growing Body*
6	*Your Health*
7	*Better Health*
8–9	*Keeping Your Health*
	(Interest levels are for students in grades 5–10)
	(Steck-Vaughn)

2.4	*First Aid Plus Biology*
2.3	*Take Care of Yourself*
	(Quercus Corporation)

4–5	*Pathways to Health Series:*
	Drugs
	Alcohol and Tobacco
	Facing the Facts
	The Pollution Problem
	Protecting our Environment
	Protecting Your Health
	Battling Disease
	Safety and First Aid
	Avoiding Accidents
	Mental Health
	Improving Your Human Relations
	Inquiry Into Consumer Education
	Getting It Together
	(Globe Book Company)

Reading Level
(Grade Equivalent)

LANGUAGE ARTS

2–8   See Random House Catalog for various books on capitalizing, punctuation, grammar, writing, vocabulary, poetry.
2.3   *Story Starters, Part 1*
4–6   *Story Starters, Part 2*
    (Steck-Vaughn Company)

1–6   *Text Extenders* (collection of paperback books of children's literature)
    Sprint Libraries: for students in grades 4–6
2.0–2.4   *Sprint Library 1–A*
2.1–2.4   *Sprint Library 1–B*
2.0–2.4   *Sprint Library 1*
2.5–2.9   *Sprint Library 2–A, 2–B, and 2*
    Scholastic Listening Skills, Unit 1
    Scholastic Listening Skills, Unit 2
    (Scholastic, Inc.)

See Garrard Publishing Company catalog for many low vocabulary books of interest to older students.

Comic book format, but well-done.   *Shakespeare: As You Like It*
    Hamlet
    Julius Caesar
    King Lear
    Macbeth
    The Merchant of Venice
    A Midsummer Night's Dream
    Othello

Reading Level
(Grade Equivalent)

Romeo and Juliet
The Taming of the Shrew
The Tempest
Twelfth Night

(Pendulum Press; Note: Each of the above is available with filmstrip and cassette.)

APPENDIX

E

A. MARSHALL HUSTON MULTISENSORY APPROACH TO LEARNING NEW READING AND SPELLING WORDS

Word cards should be prepared in advance. Words should be written in manuscript if child writes in manuscript. If child uses cursive writing, the words should be written in cursive.

Using a black magic marker, write the word on a card. Take a small bottle of Elmer's glue and go over the word with a thin line of glue. Sprinkle fine sand on the card and shake the card, making sure that all the glue is covered. Set word card aside to dry. This usually takes about five minutes.

Teaching Technique:

1. Pronounce the word.
2. Ask child to say the word.
3. Use the word in a sentence.
4. Ask the child to make up a sentence using the word.
5. Have the child act out the word. For example, if word is
   'on' - child can climb on a book, on a chair, on a box;
   'under' - child can crawl under a table, under a desk;
   'dog' - child can imitate a dog;
   'house' - child can "draw" a house in the air with his hands or pretend he is a house with his hands over his head and fingers touching at a point to illustrate the roof.

6. Demonstrate how child is to trace the word, pronouncing the word as he traces it. (Note: the *word* is pronounced as it is spoken. Do NOT sound the phonemes in isolation.) The forefinger ("pointer") should be used for tracing the word.
7. Have child trace the word *five* times, each time pronouncing the word as he traces it.
8. Turn the word card over and ask the child to write the word on a sheet of paper.
9. If child writes word correctly, proceed to Step 10; if not, repeat Step 7. (Note: child must write the entire word correctly at one time. If he bogs down, he may not look back at the word card and complete the word. He must repeat the tracing five times.)
10. Ask child to draw a picture of his new word. If new word has no concrete referral such as the word 'on', ask child to draw a picture of something *on* an object.
11. Have child write a sentence about the picture.
12. Ask child to underline the new word in his sentence, say the word, and read the entire sentence.

N O T E : This teaching technique may be used with a small group of children as well as an individual child.

GLOSSARY

alexia: refers to one who has previously been literate but has lost the ability to read as a result of acquired injury or disease to the central nervous system

ambidextrous: able to use both hands with ease for certain tasks; can do this even if one hand is considered to be the dominant or preferred hand

ambivalent use of hands: simultaneous conflicting use of the hands; no dominant (preferred) hand has been established; one hand is used just about as much as the other, sometimes referred to as *unestablished dominance*

anecdotal records: brief descriptions of specific instances of a child's behavior

antonyms: words that are opposite in meaning, such as open/shut, up/down, big/little, in/out

aniseikonia: a condition in which the lens of the eyes are not in focus; may cause readers to mix letters in words, make reversals, lose their place, and read slowly

aphasia: loss of speech

application: the ability to use a skill, a rule, a method, or some new concept in a new situation

astigmatism: an impairment of the eye that results in inability to bring the light rays to a single focal point; vision tends to be blurred and distorted, similar letters and words may be confused, sustained reading is fatiguing

audiometer: machine used to test hearing

auditory acuity: overall hearing; the sharpness or clearness of sounds transmitted to the brain

auditory discrimination: ability to discern similarities and differences among sounds

auditory dyslexia: a type of language communication disability characterized by problems in integrating and processing what is heard and recalling those sounds and applying them to the printed symbols representing them

auditory image: a mental representation (remembrance) of what has been heard

auditory memory: retention of sounds in the sequence heard

basal reader: the "textbook" (basic book) used in the teaching of reading, at successive reading levels of increasing difficulty beginning with the preprimer

Broca's area: the area of brain relating to speech function *cerebral trauma:* an injury to an area of the brain

chunking: organizing discrete units into larger meaningful units or chunks; a chunk of letters make up a word; a chunk of words form a sentence

cognitive development: the intellectual development of a child as he matures

concepts: higher and more abstract level of cognitive functioning; idea; thought; general notion

configuration: the general form or shape of a letter, word, or object

congenital: existing at or dating from birth; acquired during development in the uterus and not through heredity

context clues: method of determining the meaning of a word from other words in a passage

corrective reader: a student who has minor problems in reading which can be corrected by the classroom teacher; the services of the reading specialist are not needed

decentration: the ability to take account of several features of an object or event at the same time (Piaget)

decoding: changing the written message into a spoken message; figuring out the relationship between the writing system and the sound system

departmentalized classes: an organization of classes whereby the student moves from class to class throughout the day, changing periods and teachers according to subjects

diacritical markings: symbols used in the dictionary to designate the pronunciation of words

diagnosis: the process of identifying a disorder, such as visual or auditory dyslexia, on the basis of particular symptoms, characteristics and test patterns

diagnostic battery: a variety of standard and informal tests administered to determine specific strengths and deficiencies in different areas

dialect: a regional variety of language distinguished by features of vocabulary, grammar, and pronunciation from other regional varieties; differs from the standard form of the language

digraph: two letters which represent a single speech sound, such as the consonant digraphs *ch* in *chip, th* in *this, sh* in *shed;* or the vowel digraphs *ea* in *meat, oa* in *boat,* or *ai* in *paid*

diorama: three-dimensional picture usually constructed in a box with objects or animals placed in front of a painted background; similar to a stage with props and actors or a museum display

directionality: refers to the knowledge of left and right

disorientation: losing one's bearings; confusion as to time and space

dizygotic twins: nonidentical twins

dyslexia: a language communication disability including three general categories. The first—visual dyslexia—is characterized by reversals of letters and numerals; faulty sequencing of letters in words, numbers in series, and events in narratives; disorientation in time and space relationships and problems in processing, interpreting and recalling visual images. The second—auditory dyslexia—is characterized by problems of integrating and processing what is heard and recalling those sounds and applying them to the printed symbols representing them. The third is a combination of the two in varying degrees.

electroencephalogram (EEG): graphic record of brain waves

empathy: capacity to sense and participate in another person's feelings or ideas

etymology: the study of the origins and development of words

experience charts: charts dictated by a student or students to the teacher who acts as a scribe, recording what they have to relate about a particular happening (experience)

expressive language: writing and speaking; information emerges from a person in the form of written or spoken words to be read or heard by others

eye-hand coordination: ability of eyes and hands to work together; required for such tasks as copying or writing; sometimes referred to as visual-motor coordination

farsightedness: hyperopia (the eye is too short and the image falls behind the retina); refers to near-point vision; can affect reading and other close work

feature analysis: a process by which children recognize letters and words according to their distinctive features

finger agnosia: relative or absolute inability to show or name the fingers which have been touched, or how many fingers have been touched, in a particular test; sometimes referred to as a "short-circuit" in the neural pathways from the brain to the fingers or vice-versa

fixations: stops that the eyes make as they progress along a line of print. It is during the fixations that reading occurs.

functional literacy: the skills needed for a person to perform productively in our society

grade equivalent: the grade level representing a given score—a 5.7 is the seventh month of the fifth grade

grade level: comparable to the equivalent grade in school

hyperactivity: excessively active behavior that deviates frequently from that considered to be within a normal range

hyperopia: farsightedness (the eye is too short and the image falls behind the retina); refers to near-point vision; can affect reading and other close work

COMMON SENSE ABOUT DYSLEXIA

illiterate: as defined by the Census Bureau—someone at least 14 years old who has not completed the fifth grade

independent reading level: the level at which a student can read material with ease, understanding, and enjoyment, and without teacher assistance; sometimes called *free* or *easy reading level*

individualize: adapting instruction and materials to meet each student's individual needs, while building upon each student's individual strengths

individualized educational program (IEP): a curriculum plan which includes objectives, methodology, specific curriculum changes, and any classroom adjustments; IEPs are required by PL 94-142 for handicapped children

integration: combining of separate elements into a structured or unified whole

instructional reading level: the level used for the formal teaching of reading with basal readers; the student misses no more than five words out of a running one hundred and has a good understanding of what he reads

intelligence quotient (I.Q.): a ratio of mental ability of an individual based on performance on an intelligence test and chronological age; refers to rate of mental development

$$(I.Q. = \frac{MA}{CA} \times 100)$$

irregular words: words that are not spelled according to the way they are sounded or do not adhere to the phonics rules; sometimes called *unpredictable words*

language: a system of communication by means of spoken or written symbols (or gestures)

lateral awareness: ability to discriminate right from left

linguistic development: the development of language structure, function, and changes as a child matures

linguistics: the study of the nature and structure of language

lip movements: moving lips while silently pronouncing words to self as one reads;

long term memory: that aspect of memory that has a great capacity, lasts over a long period of time, and has organized or chunked information into patterns

mainstreaming: placing dyslexic or other handicapped children in regular classes and integrating them into the regular school program while receiving support from special teachers

maturation: those aspects of development which are a part of the biological make-up of a child, and which inevitably will occur if the child's environment is reasonably appropriate

248

maturational lag: a late development of areas of the brain controlling certain perceptual and motor functions

mnemonic device: something used to help in remembering

monozygotic twins: identical twins (single-ovum)

motivation: interest, drive, incentive to do something; intrinsic motivation comes from within, extrinsic from outside as a result of rewards or punishments

mutant: produced by mutation, a change in hereditary material

myelin sheath: the fatty substance that covers the axon, along which nerve impulses travel

myopia: nearsightedness (the eye is too long and the image falls in front of the retina); refers to far-point vision; can affect reading correctly from the chalkboard, charts, or an overhead projector

nearsightedness: myopia: (the eye is too long and the image falls in front of the retina); refers to far-point vision; can affect reading correctly from the chalkboard, charts, or an overhead projector

negative transfer: a term used to indicate when a child has been taught something a certain way, then has to "unlearn" it, and learn it again

occipital lobe: area of brain concerned with vision

open classroom: an organization of classes whereby large groups of students work in large central areas with several teachers; a decentralized classroom arrangement

oral reinforcement: saying the words softly to one's self as one reads

orthography: way of writing; the letters of our alphabet (Aa, Bb, Cc) are a form of orthography

parietal lobe: area of brain concerned with visual association

phonological shifts: developmental shifts in speech sounds and changes of sounds as children mature

polygenic: a group of nonallelic genes that collectively control the inheritance of a quantitative character or modify the expression of a qualitative character

positive reinforcement: the strengthening of a response by an encouraging comment, action, or reward

practical charts: charts prepared especially for teaching the new vocabulary in basal reader stories

preprimer: first "formal" book used in the teaching of reading

prerequisite knowledge: the readiness necessary to acquire new learnings; the basic understandings, skills, knowledge that serve as the foundation and springboard for information to be learned

problem solving: using thinking to combine principles and obtain new solutions

process: continuous actions or operations toward an end, as the *reading process processing:* the handling of information by a series of active steps

readability: the difficulty of reading material

reading level: the level at which a child is reading, usually expressed in terms of grade level. A student in the fourth grade may have a reading level of fourth grade, third grade, or fifth grade; that is, lower or higher than the school grade in which he is placed

reading readiness: the basic understandings, skills, and maturational development that serve as the foundation and bridge into formal reading instruction; can also apply to the reading of textbooks as one moves up through the grades

reading retardation: reading performance significantly below one's ability to read.

reauditorize: to remember and "hear" in one's mind the sound of something one has heard

recall: the remembrance of what has been seen or heard (or experienced in another way)

receptive language: reading and listening; that which is read and heard, and filters into the brain for processing

regressive eye movements: a shift of the eye to the left along a line of print to return to a word or words to get another look

reliability: the degree to which a test gives consistent results

remedial reader: a student who is not reading according to his ability and whose achievement and difficulties are such that he needs special help by the reading specialist in addition to what he receives in his regular classroom

retention: learning that permits later recall or recognition

return sweep: the diagonal sweep of the eyes from the end of a line of print to begin reading on the next line of print

reversals: changing the position or orientation of numbers, letters, parts of a word, or words, such as 6 for 9, *d* for *b, w* for *m, iorn* for *iron*, or *was* for *saw*

revisualize: to remember and "picture" in one's mind something one has seen

round-robin teaching: refers to the practice of having children take turns reading orally from the basal reader (or textbook); sometimes called the "next, next" procedure

saccades: jerky movements of the eyes along a line of print

schwa: a softened, unaccented vowel sound; represented by the symbol ə; the vowel sound *a* in *a*bout, the *o* in butt*o*n; any of the vowels may represent the schwa sound in certain words

self-concept: how a child views himself and how he perceives others see him

semantical shifts: developmental shifts in the relations between referents and names, and concepts and names, as children mature *sequencing:* placing ideas, events, letters, and words in logical or chronological order, and numbers in a certain numerical order

short-term memory: that aspect of memory that is limited in capacity, lasts only briefly, and has rapid input and output; sometimes called our working memory

sight-vocabulary: stock of words which a child can recognize instantly without having to resort to the application of word recognition strategies

space: the three-dimensional extension in which objects and events exist, occur, and have relative position and direction

specialized vocabulary: words indigenous to particular subject matter, such as those used in science, social studies or math

spoonerism: a transposition of initial sounds of two or more words, such as *sons* of *toil* for *tons* of *soil*; a characteristic of auditory dyslexia

standardized test: a test with specific procedures and certain tasks, and for which norms have been established so that comparable measurements may be obtained in different geographical regions

strabismus: muscular imbalance resulting from an incoordination of the muscles that move the eyeball; can cause omission of letters, losing place on line, displacement of words

strephosymbolia: "twisted symbols" as in reversing *no* and *on* or *saw* and *was* (coined by Dr. Samuel Orton)

syndrome: a cluster of symptoms or characteristics which together indicate a disorder

syntactical shifts: developmental shifts in grammatical relations as children mature

tachistoscope: a mechanical device that rapidly exposes reading material at differing rates of exposure

telebinocular: machine used to test vision

traditional self-contained classroom: a classroom where students are with the same teacher for the entire day and where the teacher teaches the different subjects to the class

transfer of learning: learning a concept, skill or understanding in one situation and being able to apply it in another; learning one thing helps in learning something else

transposition: a change in sequence of letters (or sounds) within a word, such as *iorn* for *iron* or *emeny* for *enemy*; or words in a phrase or sentence, such as *gray, little fox* for *little, gray fox*

unpredictable words: words that are not spelled according to the way they are sounded, or do not adhere to the phonics rules; sometimes called *irregular words*

validity: the extent to which a test represents a balanced and adequate sampling of the instructional outcomes it is intended to cover

visual acuity: refers to overall vision; the sharpness or clearness of a visual image transmitted to the brain

visual discrimination: the ability to discern similarities and differences in letters and words when looking at them

visual dyslexia: a type of language communication disability characterized by reversals of letters and numerals; faulty sequencing of letters in words, numbers in series, and events in narrative; disorientation in time and space relationships; and problems in processing, interpreting and recalling visual images

visual image: a mental representation (remembrance) of what has been seen

visual memory: the retention of objects, events, or words seen

visual-motor coordination: ability of the hands and eyes to work together, sometimes called eye-hand coordination; required for such tasks as copying or writing

word banks: a file of known words which a student selects from his own stories or language experience charts

word-blindness: a term formerly used to indicate the inability to read words as a result of congenital or acquired causes

BIBLIOGRAPHY

Aaron, Ira E., "Translating research into practice: Reading readiness, visual perception, and auditory perception," in Helen K. Smith, ed., *Perception and Reading* (Newark, Delaware: International Reading Association, 1968), pp. 130–135.

Aaron, P. G., "The neuropsychology of developmental dyslexia," in R. N. Malatesha and P. G. Aaron, eds., *Reading Disorders, Varieties and Treatments* (New York: Academic Press, 1982), pp. 5–67.

Aaron, P. G., and Bakes, Catherine, "Empirical and heuristic bases for diagnosis and remediation of specific reading disabilities," *Topics in Learning and Learning Disabilities: Issues in Reading Diagnosis* Vol. 2, No. 4. (Gaithersburg, Pa.: Aspen Systems, January, 1983).

Adams, Richard B., "Dyslexia: A discussion of its definition," *Journal of Learning Disabilities* 2 (December 1969), pp. 616–626.

Adler, Mortimer J., and Van Doren, Charles, *How to Read A Book* (Simon and Schuster, 1972).

Adler, Mortimer, *How to Speak, How to Listen* (New York: Macmillan, 1983).

Anderson, Paul S., ed., *Linguistics in the Elementary School Classroom* (New York: Macmillan, 1971).

Atteberry, Mary Wade, "Dyslexia, do its 'victims' have unusual ability?" *The Indianapolis Star* (Nov. 4, 1984), Section F, pp. 1–2.

Auten, Anne, "The ultimate connection: Reading, listening, writing, speaking, thinking," *The Reading Teacher* Vol. 36, No. 6 (February 1983), pp. 584–587.

Bader, Lois A., *Reading Diagnosis and Remediation in Classroom and Clinic* (New York: Macmillan, 1980).

Baker, Ray Stannard, *Woodrow Wilson, Life and Letters Youth 1856–1890* (Garden City, New York: Doubleday, Page and Co., 1927).

Bakker, Dirk J. and Satz, Paul, eds., *Specific Reading Disability: Advances in Theory and Method* (The Netherlands: Rotterdam University Press, 1970).

Balajthy, Ernest, "Reinforcement and drill by microcomputer," *The Reading Teacher* Vol. 37, No. 6 (February 1984), pp. 490–494.

Bannatyne, Alexander, *Language, Reading and Learning Disabilities* (Springfield, Illinois: Charles C. Thomas, 1971).

Barnett, Lincoln, "The English language," in Hal D. Funk and DeWayne Triplett, eds., *Language Arts in the Elementary School: Readings* (Philadelphia: Lippincott, 1972), pp. 95–103.

Bateman, Barbara, *Learning Disorders, Reading* Vol. 4 (Seattle, Washington: Special Child Publications, 1971).

Baumann, James F., and Stevenson, Jennifer A., "Understanding standardized reading achievement test scores," *The Reading Teacher* Vol. 35, No. 6 (March 1982), pp. 648–654.

Beers, Carol S., "The relationship of cognitive development to spelling and reading abilities," in Edmund H. Henderson and James W. Beers, eds., *Developmental and Cognitive Aspects of Learning to Spell: A Reflection of Word Knowledge* (Newark, Delaware: International Reading Association, 1980), pp. 74–84.

Beers, James W., "Developmental strategies of spelling competence in primary school children," in Edmund H. Henderson and James W. Beers, eds., *Developmental and Cognitive Aspects of Learning to Spell: A Reflection of Word Knowledge* (Newark, Delaware: International Reading Association, 1980), pp. 36–45.

Beers, James W., and Edmund H. Henderson, "A study of developing orthographic concepts among first graders," *Research in the Teaching of English* 11 (Fall 1977), pp. 133–148.

Beery, Keith E., *Monograph: Visual-Motor Integration* (Chicago: Follett Publications, 1967).

Benirschke, Kurt, "Accurate recording of twin placentation, a plea to the obstetrician," *Obstetrics and Gynecology* Vol. 18 (September 1961), pp. 334–347.

Benton, Arthur L., "Dyslexia in relation to form perception and directional sense," in John Money, ed., *Reading Disability, Progress and Research Needs in Dyslexia*, (Baltimore: The Johns Hopkins Press, 1962), pp. 81–102.

_____, "Right-left discrimination, *Pediatric Clinics of North America* 15 (1968), pp. 747–758.

_____, *Right-Left Discrimination and Finger Localization* (New York: Harper and Brothers, 1959).

_____, "Significance of systematic reversal in right-left discrimination," *Acta Psychological et Neurological* Vol. 33 (1957), pp. 129–137.

Benton, Arthur L., and Pearl, David, eds., *Dyslexia: An Appraisal of Current Knowledge* (New York: Oxford University Press, 1978).

Blue, Rose, *Me and Einstein* (New York: Human Sciences, 1979).

Blumenson, Martin, *The Patton Papers.* Vols I and II. (Boston: Houghton Mifflin, 1974).

Boder, Elena, "Developmental dyslexia: A diagnostic approach based on three atypical reading-spelling patterns," *Developmental Medicine and Child Neurology* 15 (1973) pp. 663–687.

_____, "Developmental dyslexia: A diagnostic screening procedure based on three characteristic patterns of reading and spelling," in Barbara Bateman, ed., *Learning Disorders, Reading* Vol. 4 (1971) (Seattle, Wash.: Special Child Publications), pp. 297–342.

_____, "Developmental dyslexia, a new diagnostic approach based on the identification of three subtypes," *The Journal of School Health* Vol. 40, No. 6 (June 1970), pp. 289–290.

_____, "Developmental dyslexia: Prevailing diagnostic concepts and a new diagnostic approach," in Helmer R. Myklebust, ed., *Progress in Learning Disabilities* Vol. II (New York: Grune and Stratton, 1971), pp. 293–321.

Bond, Guy L., Tinker, Miles A., Wasson, Barbara B., and Wasson, John B., *Reading Difficulties, Their Diagnosis and Correction,* 5th ed. (Englewood Cliffs, New Jersey: Prentice-Hall, 1984).

Boyd, Gertrude A., *Teaching Communication Skills in the Elementary School* (New York: Van Nostrand Reinhold, 1970).

Brander, T., cited by Edith Zerbin-Rubin in "Congenital word-blindness," *Bulletin of the Orton Society* Vol. 17 (1967), pp. 47–54.

Broadbent, Sir William Henry, "On the cerebral mechanism of speech and thought," *Medico-Chirurgical Transactions* Vol. 37 (London: The Royal Medical and Chirurgical Society of London, Longmans, Green, Reader, and Dyer, 1872), pp. 145–194.

_____, "Note on Dr. Hinshelwood's communication on word-blindness and visual memory," *The Lancet* (January 4, 1896), p. 18.

Brown, Don A., *Reading Diagnosis and Remediation* (Englewood Cliffs, New Jersey: Prentice-Hall, 1982).

Burg, Leslie, and Kaufman, Maurice, "Laws about special education: Their impact on the use of reading specialists," *The Reading Teacher* Vol. 34, No. 2 (November 1980), pp. 187–191.

Burns, Paul C., Roe, Betty D., and Ross, Elinor P., *Teaching Reading in Today's Elementary Schools* (Boston: Houghton Mifflin, 1984).

Burns, Paul G., and Broman, Betty L., *The Language Arts in Childhood Education* 4th ed. (Chicago: Rand McNally, 1979).

Calder, Ritchie, *Leonardo and the Age of the Eye* (New York: Simon and Schuster, 1970).

Caldarelli, David D. and Campanella, Ruth S., "Ear," *The World Book Encyclopedia*, Vol. 6 (1985), pp. 5–8.

Carlson, Thorsten, ed., *Administrators and Reading* (New York: Harcourt Brace Jovanovich, 1972).

Carlton, Lessie and Moore, Robert H., *Reading, Self-Directive Dramatization and Self-Concept* (Columbus, Ohio: Charles E. Merrill, 1968).

Chalfant, James C., and Flathouse, Virgil E., "Auditory and visual learning," in Helmer R. Myklebust, ed., *Progress in Learning Disabilities* Vol. II (New York: Grune and Stratton, 1971), pp. 252–292.

Chomsky, Carol, "Reading, writing and phonology," *Harvard Educational Review* Vol. 40 (May 1970), pp. 287–309.

_____, "Write first, read later," *Childhood Education* Vol. 47 (March 1971), pp. 296–299.

Chomsky, Noam and Halle, Morris, *The Sound Patterns of English* (New York: Harper and Row, 1968).

Cohen, Elizabeth G., Intilli, Jo-Ann K., and Robbins, Susan Hurevitz, "Teachers and reading specialists: Cooperation or isolation?" *The Reading Teacher* Vol. 32, No. 3 (December 1978), pp. 281–287.

Collins-Cheek, Martha, and Cheek, Earl H., Jr., *Diagnostic-Prescriptive Reading Instruction, A Guide for Classroom Teachers* (Dubuque, Iowa: Wm. C. Brown, 1984).

Cranston, Ruth, *The Story of Woodrow Wilson* (New York: Simon and Schuster, 1945).

Criqui, Orvel A., "An administrator's view of reading programs," *The Reading Teacher* Vol. 30, No. 4 (January 1977), pp. 356–358.

Crisculolo, Nicholas P., "Effective ways to communicate with parents about reading," *The Reading Teacher* Vol. 34, No. 2 (November 1980), pp. 164–166.

Critchley, Macdonald, *The Dyslexic Child* (Springfield, Illinois: Charles C. Thomas, 1970).

_____, "Some problems of the ex-dyslexic," *Bulletin of the Orton Society* Vol. 23 (1973), pp. 7–14.

Critchley, Macdonald, and Critchley, Eileen A., *Dyslexia Defined* (Springfield, Illinois: Charles C. Thomas, 1978).

Cronnel, Bruce, "Phonics for reading vs. phonics for spelling," *The Reading Teacher* Vol. 32, No. 3 (December 1978), pp. 337–340.

Crosby, Robert M. N., "Reading: The dyslexic child," *Today's Education* Vol. 60, No. 7 (October 1971), pp. 46–48.

Cunningham, Pat, "Horizontal reading," *The Reading Teacher* Vol. 34, No. 2 (November 1980), pp. 222–224.

Dallman, Martha, Rouch, Roger L., Char, Lynette Y.C., and DeBoer, John J., *The Teaching of Reading*, 6th ed. (New York: Holt, Rinehart and Winston, 1982).

Daniels, Josephus, *The Life of Woodrow Wilson* (Chicago: John C. Winston, 1924).

Dauzat, Jo Ann, and Dauzat, Sam V., *Reading: The Teacher and the Learner* (New York: John Wiley and Sons, 1981).

Dechant, Emerald, *Diagnosis and Remediation of Reading Disabilities* (Englewood Cliffs, New Jersey: Prentice-Hall, 1981).

_____, *Improving the Teaching of Reading* (Englewood Cliffs, New Jersey: Prentice-Hall, 1970).

Decker, Sadie N., and DeFries, J.C., "Cognitive abilities in families with reading disabled children," *Journal of Learning Disabilities* Vol. 13, No. 9 (1980), pp. 53–57.

DeFries, J. C., and Decker, S. N., "Genetic aspects of reading disability: A family study" in R. N. Malatesha and P. G. Aaron, eds., *Reading Disorders, Varieties and Treatments* (New York: Academic Press, 1982), pp. 255–279.

DeStefano, Johanna S., and Fox, Sharon E., *Language and the Language Arts* (Boston: Little, Brown, 1974).

DiStefano, Philip P., and Hagerty, Patricia J., "Teaching spelling at the elementary level: A realistic perspective," *The Reading Teacher* Vol. 38 (January 1985), pp. 373–377.

Doehring, Donald G., *Patterns of Impairment in Specific Reading Disability* (Bloomington, Indiana: Indiana University Press, 1968).

Doehring, Donald G., Trites, Ronald L., Patel, P. G., and Fiedorowicz, A.M., *Reading Disabilities, The Interaction of Reading, Language, and Neuropsychological Deficits* (New York: Academic Press, 1981).

Downing, John, *Comparative Reading, Cross-National Studies of Behavior and Processes in Reading and Writing* (New York: Macmillan, 1973).

Duane, Drake D., "A neurologic overview of specific language disability for the non-neurologist," *Bulletin of the Orton Society* Vol. 24 (1974), pp. 5–36.

Duane, Drake D., and Rome, Paula Dozier, eds., *The Dyslexic Child* (New York: Insight Publishing, 1979).

Duane, Drake D. and Rawson, Margaret B., eds., *Reading, Perception and Language*, papers from the World Congress on Dyslexia (Baltimore: York, 1974).

Dunn, Rita, "Learning style and its relation to exceptionality at both ends of the spectrum," *Exceptional Children* Vol. 49, No. 6 (April 1983), pp. 496–506.

"Dyslexia, The Hidden Handicap," special educational needs report of the Committee of Enquiry into the education of handicapped children and young people (Peppard, Oxfordshire: British Dyslexia Association, n.d.).

Edwards, R. Philip, Alley, Gordon R., and Snider, William, "Academic achievement and minimal brain dysfunction," *Journal of Learning Disabilities* Vol. 4, No. 3 (March 1971), pp. 17–21.

Ekwall, Eldon E., *Diagnosis and Remediation of the Disabled Reader* (Boston: Allyn and Bacon, 1976).

_____, *Locating and Correcting Reading Difficulties*, 4th ed. (Columbus, Ohio: Charles E. Merrill, 1985).

_____, ed., *Psychological Factors in the Teaching of Reading* (Columbus, Ohio: Charles E. Merrill, 1973).

Ekwall, Eldon E., and Shanker, James L., *Teaching Reading in the Elementary School* (Columbus, Ohio: Charles E. Merrill, 1985).

Elkind, David, *Children and Adolescents Interpretive Essays on Jean Piaget*, 2nd ed. (New York: Oxford University Press, 1974).

Elkind, David, Horn, John, and Schneider, Gerrie, "Modified word recognition, reading achievement and perceptual de-centration," *The Journal of Genetic Psychology* Vol. 107 (December 1965), pp. 235–251.

Ellis, Andrew W., *Reading, Writing and Dyslexia: A Cognitive Analysis* (Hillsdale, New Jersey: Lawrence Erlbaum Association, 1984).

Evans, James R., "Neuropsychologically based remedial reading procedures: Some possibilities," in R. N. Malatesha and P. G. Aaron, eds., *Reading Disorders, Varieties and Treatments* (New York: Academic Press, 1982), pp. 371–388.

Evans, James S., *An Uncommon Gift* (Philadelphia: Westminister Press, 1983).

Evans, Martha M., *Dyslexia, An Annotated Bibliography* (Westport, Connecticut: Greenwood Press, 1982).

Farago, Ladislas, *Patton: Ordeal and Triumph* (New York: Dell, 1963).

Farr, Roger, and Roser, Nancy, *Teaching A Child To Read* (New York: Harcourt Brace Jovanovich, 1979).

Fernald, Grace, *Remedial Techniques in Basic School Subjects* (New York: McGraw-Hill, 1971/1943).

Finucci, Joan M., "Genetic considerations in dyslexia," in Helmer R. Myklebust, ed., *Progress in Learning Disabilities* Vol. IV (1978) (New York: Grune and Stratton), pp. 41–63.

Finucci, Joan M., Guthrie, John T., Childs, Anne L., Abbey, Helen, and Childs, Barton, "The genetics of specific reading disability," *Annals of Human Genetics* 40 (1976), London, p. 1–23.

Fleming, Elizabeth, *Believe the Heart* (San Francisco, California: Strawberry Hill, 1984).

Frauenheim, John G., "Academic achievement characteristics of adult males who were diagnosed as dyslexic in childhood," *Journal of Learning Disabilities* Vol. 11, No. 8 (October 1978), pp. 21–28.

Frith, Uta, and Frith, Christopher, "Relationships between reading and spelling," in James F. Kavanagh and Richard L. Venezky, eds., *Orthography, Reading, and Dyslexia* (Baltimore: University Park Press, 1980), pp. 287–295.

Funk, Hal D., and Triplett, DeWayne, *Language Arts in the Elementary School: Readings* (Philadelphia: J.B. Lippincott, 1972).

Furth, Hans G., *Piaget for Teachers* (Englewood Cliffs, New Jersey: Prentice-Hall, 1970).

Gaddes, William H., *Learning Disabilities and Brain Function, A Neuropsychological Approach* (New York: Springer-Verlag, 1980).

Galaburda, Albert M., and Kemper, Thomas L., "Cytoarchitectonic abnormalities in developmental dyslexia: A case study," *Annals of Neurology* Vol. 6 (August 1979), pp. 94–100.

Gambrell, Linda B., "Dialogue journals: Reading-writing interaction," *The Reading Teacher* Vol. 38 (February 1985), pp. 512–515.

_____, "Think-time: Implications for reading instruction," *The Reading Teacher* Vol. 34, No. 2 (November 1980), pp. 143–146.

Gamby, Gert, "Talking books and taped books: Materials for instruction," *The Reading Teacher* Vol. 36, No. 4 (January 1983), pp. 366–369.

Gentry, J. Richard, "An analysis of developmental spelling in GNYS AT WRK," *The Reading Teacher* Vol. 36, No. 2 (November 1982), pp. 191–192.

_____, "Learning to spell developmentally," *The Reading Teacher* Vol. 34, No. 4 (January 1981), pp.378–381.

Geschwind, Norman, Galaburda, Albert and LeMay, Marjorie, "Morphological and physiological substrates of language and cognitive development," in Robert Katzman, ed., *Congenital and Acquired Cognitive Disorders* (New York: Raven Press, 1979), pp. 31–41.

Gillespi-Silver, Patricia, *Teaching Reading to Children with Special Needs*, (Columbus, Ohio: Charles E. Merril, 1979).

Gillet, Jean Wallace, and Temple, Charles, *Understanding Reading Problems, Assessment and Instruction* (Boston: Little, Brown and Company, 1982).

Goldberg, Herman K., Schiffman, Gilbert B., and Bender, Michael, *Dyslexia, Interdisciplinary Approaches to Reading Disabilities* (New York: Grune and Stratton, 1983).

Goldberg, Herman K., and Schiffman, Gilbert B., *Dyslexia Problems of Reading Disabilities* (New York: Grune and Stratton, 1972).

Goldberg, Morton F., "Eye," *The World Book Encyclopedia*, Vol. 6 (1985), pp. 358–367.

Goodman, Kenneth S., and Fleming, James T., eds., *Psycholinguistics and the Teaching of Reading,* selected papers from the IRA Pre-Convention Institute held in Boston, April 1968. (Newark, Delaware: International Reading Association, 1972).

Gosse, Edmund, "Andersen, Hans Christian," *The Encyclopedia Britannica,* 11th ed., Vol. 1 (1911), pp. 958–959.

Gottfredson, Linda S., Finucci, Joan M., and Childs, Barton, "The adult occupational success of dyslexic boys: A large scale, long-term follow up," Report No. 334 (March 1983) (Baltimore: The Center for Social Organization of Schools at The Johns Hopkins University).

Gow, David W., "Dyslexic adolescent boys: Classroom remediation is not enough," *Bulletin of the Orton Society* Vol. 24 (1974), pp. 154–163.

Grabe, Mark, and Grabe, Cindy. "The microcomputer and the language experience approach," *The Reading Teacher* Vol. 38 (February 1985), pp. 508 511.

Granschow, Leonore, "Analyze error patterns to remediate severe spelling difficulties," *The Reading Teacher* Vol. 38 (December 1984), pp. 288–293.

Graves, Donald H., *Writing: Teachers and Children at Work* (Exeter, New Hampshire: Heinemann Educational Books, 1983).

Griffiths, Anita N., *Teaching the Dyslexic Child* (Novato, California: Academic Therapy, 1978).

Gunning, Thomas G., "Wrong level test: Wrong information," *The Reading Teacher* Vol. 35, No. 8 (May 1982), pp. 902–905.

Guthrie, John T., "Research views: Classroom management," *The Reading Teacher* Vol. 36, No. 6 (February 1983), pp. 606–608.

Hall, Mary Anne, *Teaching Reading as a Language Experience* (Columbus, Ohio: Charles E. Merrill, 1981).

Hallgren, Bertil, *Specific Dyslexia ("Congenital Word-Blindness"); A Clinical and Genetic Study* (Copenhagen: Ejnar Munksgaard, 1950. Translated from the Swedish by Erica Odelberg. (Stockholm: Esseite aktiebolag, 1950).

Harris, Albert J., and Sipay, Edward R., *How to Increase Reading Ability*, 7th ed. (New York: Longman Press, 1980).

_____, *How to Teach Reading* (New York: Longman Press, 1979).

_____, *Readings on Reading Instruction*, 3rd ed. (New York: Longman Press, 1984).

Harris, Larry A., and Smith, Carl B., *Reading Instruction, Diagnostic Teaching in the Classroom*, 3rd ed. (New York: Holt, Rinehart and Winston, 1980).

Heilman, Arthur W., *Phonics in Proper Perspective*, 5th ed. (Columbus, Ohio: Charles E. Merrill, 1985).

Heilman, Arthur W., Blair, Timothy R., and Rupley, William H., *Principles and Practices of Teaching Reading*, 5th ed. (Columbus, Ohio: Charles E. Merrill, 1981).

Henderson, Edmund H., and Beers, James W., eds., *Developmental and Cognitive Aspects of Learning to Spell, A Reflection of Word Knowledge* (Newark, Delaware: International Reading Association, 1980).

Hermann, Knud, *Reading Disability, A Medical Study of Word-Blindness and Related Handicaps* (Springfield, Illinois: Charles C. Thomas, 1959).

Herrick, Virgil E., "Children's experiences in writing," in Virgil E. Herrick and Leland B. Jacobs, eds., *Children and the Language Arts* (Englewood Cliffs, New Jersey: Prentice-Hall, 1955), pp. 271–272.

Hillerich, Robert, "Let's teach spelling—not phonetic misspelling," *Language Arts* Vol. 54 (March 1977), pp. 301–307.

Hinshelwood, James, "A case of dyslexia: A peculiar form of word-blindness," *The Lancet* (Nov. 21, 1896), pp. 1451–1454.

_____, "A case of 'word' without 'letter' blindness," *The Lancet* (Feb. 12, 1898), pp. 422–425.

_____, "Congenital word-blindness," *The Lancet* (May 26, 1900), pp. 1506–1508.

_____, "Congenital Word-Blindness (London: H.K. Lewis, 1917).

_____, " 'Letter' without 'word' blindness," *The Lancet* (Jan. 14, 1899), pp. 85–86.

_____, *Letter-, Word-, and Mind-Blindness* (London: H.K. Lewis, 1900).

_____, "Word-blindness and visual memory," *The Lancet* (Dec. 21, 1895), pp. 1564–1570.

Hochberg, Julian. "Attention in perception and reading," in Francis A. Young and Donald B. Lindsley, eds., *Early Experience and Visual Information Processing in Perceptual and Reading Disorders* (Washington, D.C.: National Academy of Sciences, 1970), pp. 219–224.

Horn, Ernest, "Spelling," *Encyclopedia of Educational Research*, 3rd ed. (New York: Macmillan, 1960), p. 1337

Hornsby, Bevé, *Overcoming Dyslexia* (New York: Arco, 1984).

Huey, Edmund Burke, *The Psychology and Pedagogy of Reading* (Cambridge, Mass.: The M.I.T. Press, 1908/1968).

Hughs, John R., "The electroencephalogram and reading disorders," in R. N. Malatesha and P. G. Aaron, eds., *Reading Disorders, Varieties and Treatments* (New York: Academic Press, 1982), pp. 234–253.

Ingram, T. T. S., Mason, A.W., and Blackburn, J., "A retrospective study of 82 children with reading disability," *Developmental Medicine and Child Neurology* 12 (1970), pp. 271–281.

Ingram, Thomas T. S., "The nature of dyslexia," in Francis A. Young and Donald B. Lindsley, eds., *Early Experience and Visual Information Processing in Perceptual and Reading Disorders* (Washington, D.C.: National Academy of Sciences, 1970), pp. 405–444.

Jacob, Stanley W., Francone, Clarice Ashworth, and Lossow, Walter J., *Structure and Function in Man*, 4th ed. (Philadelphia: W.B. Saunders, 1978).

Jansky, Jeannette, and De Hirsch, Katrina, *Preventing Reading Failure: Prediction, Diagnosis, Intervention* (New York: Harper and Row, 1972).

Jenkins, R.L., Brown, A. W., and Elmerdorf, L., "Mixed dominance and reading disability," as cited in Edith Zerbin-Rubin, "Congenital word-blindness," *Bulletin of the Orton Society* Vol. 17 (1967), pp. 47–54.

Johnson, Doris J., and Myklebust, Helmer R., *Learning Disabilities, Educational Principles and Practices* (New York: Grune and Stratton, 1967).

Jordan, Dale R., *Dyslexia in the Classroom*, 2nd ed. (Columbus, Ohio: Charles E. Merrill, 1977).

Kaluger, George, and Kolson, Clifford J., *Reading and Learning Disabilities* (Columbus, Ohio: Charles E. Merrill, 1978).

Karlin, Robert, *Teaching Elementary Reading, Principles and Strategies*, 3rd ed. (New York: Harcourt Brace Jovanovich, 1980).

Katzman, Robert ed., *Congenital and Acquired Cognitive Disorders* (New York: Raven Press, 1979).

Kavanagh, James F., and Mattingly, Ignatius G., eds., *Language by Ear and by Eye* (Cambridge, Mass.: The M.I.T. Press, 1972).

Kavanagh, James F., and Venezky, Richard L., *Orthography, Reading and Dyslexia* (Baltimore: University Park Press, 1980).

Kerr, James, "School hygiene, in its mental, moral, and physical aspects," *Journal of the Royal Statistical Society* 60 (1897), pp. 613–680.

Kinsbourne, Marcel, "Developmental gerstmann syndrome," *Pediatric Clinics of North America* Vol. 15, No. 3 (August 1968), pp. 771–777.

_____, "Prospects for the study of developmental reading backwardness," *The British Journal of Disorders of Communication* Vol. 2, No. 2 (1967), pp. 152–154.

_____, "The analysis of learning deficit with special reference to selective attention," in Dirk J. Bakker and Paul Satz, eds., *Specific Reading Disability: Advances in Theory and Method* (The Netherlands: Rotterdam University Press, 1970), pp. 115–122.

_____, "The role of selective attention in reading disability," in P. G. Aaron and R. N. Malatesha, eds., *Reading Disorders, Varieties and Treatments* (New York: Academic Press, 1982), pp. 199–214.

Klasen, Edith, *The Syndrome of Specific Dyslexia* (Baltimore: University Park Press, 1972).

Kolers, Paul A., "Three stages of reading," in Harry Levin and Joanna Williams, eds., *Basic Studies in Reading* (New York: Basic Books,

1970), pp. 90–118. Also in Frank Smith ed., *Psycholinguistics and Reading* (New York: Holt, Rinehart and Winston, 1973).

Koppitz, Elizabeth M., *The Bender Gestalt Test for Young Children* (New York: Grune and Stratton, 1971).

Larrick, Nancy, *A Parent's Guide to Children's Reading*, 4th ed. (New York: Bantam Books, 1975).

Lehr, Fran, "Grade repetition vs. social promotion," *The Reading Teacher* Vol. 36, No. 2 (November 1982), pp. 234–237.

Lenkowsky, Linda Klein, and Saposnek, Donald T., "Family consequences of parental dyslexia," *Journal of Learning Disabilities* Vol. 11, No. 1 (January 1978), pp. 59–65.

Lerner, Janet W., *Children With Learning Disabilities* (Boston: Houghton Mifflin, 1971).

_____, "Remedial reading and learning disabilities: Are they the same or different?" *Journal of Special Education* Vol. 9 (Feb. 19, 1975), pp. 119–131.

Levin, Harry, and Joanna P. Williams, eds., *Basic Studies on Reading* (New York: Basic Books, 1970).

Levinson, Harold N., *A Solution to the Riddle Dyslexia* (New York: Springer-Verlag, 1980).

_____, *Smart But Feeling Dumb* (New York: Warner Books, 1984).

Ley, J., and Tordeur, G.W., "Alexie et agraphie d'évolution chez des jumeaux monozygotiques," *Journal Belgium Neurological Psychiatry* 36 (1936), p. 102, as cited in Edith Zerbin-Rubin, "Congenital word-blindness," *Bulletin of the Orton Society* Vol. 17 (1967), pp. 47–54.

Liberman, Alvin M., "General discussion of Templin's study of articulation and language development during the early school years," in Frank Smith and George A. Miller, eds., *The Genesis of Language, A Psycholinguistic Approach* (Cambridge, Mass.: The M.I.T. Press, 1966).

Link, Arthur S., *Wilson, The Road to the White House* (Princeton, New Jersey: Princeton University Press, 1947).

Linksz, Arthur, *On Writing, Reading, and Dyslexia* (New York: Grune and Stratton, 1973).

Loban, Walter, "What language reveals," in James B. MacDonald and Robert R. Leeper, eds., *Language and Meaning* (Washington, D.C.: Association for Supervision and Curriculum Development, 1966), p. 73.

Loomer, Bradley M., "Educator's guide to spelling research and practice" (Des Moines, Iowa: Iowa State Department of Public Instruction, Iowa City, Iowa: University of Iowa, 1978), pp. 1–33.

Losen, Stuart M. and Losen, Joyce Garskof, *The Special Education Team* (Boston: Allyn and Bacon, 1985).

Malatesha, R. N., and Dougan, Deborah R., "Clinical subtypes of developmental dyslexia," in R. N. Malatesha and P. G. Aaron, eds., *Reading Disorders, Varieties and Treatments* (New York: Academic Press, 1982), pp. 69–92.

Malmstrom, Jean, *Understanding Language, A Primer for the Language Arts Teacher* (New York: St. Martin's Press, 1977).

Marain, S. Donald, ed., *Human Development and Reading Instruction* (Cambridge, Mass.: Educators Publishing, 1977).

Masland, Richard L., "The advantages of being dyslexic," *Bulletin of the Orton Society* Vol. 26 (1976), pp. 10–18.

Mason, George E., "The computer in the reading clinic," *The Reading Teacher* Vol. 36, No. 6 (February 1983), pp. 504–506.

_____, "The word processor and teaching reading," *The Reading Teacher* Vol. 37, No. 6 (February 1984), pp. 552–553.

Martin, Reed, "The teacher's rights in PL. 94-142," editor's interview, "A Conversation with Attorney Reed Martin," *Journal of Learning Disabilities* Vol. 2 (June/July 1978), pp. 4–14.

Massaro, Dominic V., ed., *Understanding Language, An Information-Processing Analysis of Speech Perception, Reading, and Psycholinguistics* (New York: Academic Press, 1975).

Matejek, Zdenek with Rawson, Margaret B., "Dyslexia, an international problem: A report from Czechoslovakia," *Bulletin of the Orton Society* 15 (1965), pp. 24–30.

McCarthy, James J., and McCarthy, Joan F., *Learning Disabilities* (Boston: Allyn and Bacon, 1969).

McClelland, Jane, "Adolescents: It's never too late to learn," *Bulletin of the Orton Society* Vol. 24 (1974), pp. 141–153.

McNeil, John D., *Reading Comprehension, New Directions for Classroom Practice* (Glenview, Illinois: Scott, Foresman, Inc., 1984).

McWilliams, John R., "Eye," *The World Book Encyclopedia* Vol. 6 (1969) (Chicago, Illinois: Field Enterprises Educational Corp.), pp. 357–363.

Mencken, H. L., *The American Language, An Inquiry Into the Development of English in the United States* (New York: Alfred A. Knopf, 1980).

Menyuk, Paula, *Language and Maturation* (Cambridge, Mass.: The M.I.T. Press, 1977).

_____, *The Acquisition and Development of Language* (Englewood Cliffs, New Jersey: Prentice-Hall, 1971).

Mercer, Cecil D., *Students With Learning Disabilities* (Columbus, Ohio: Charles E. Merrill, 1983).

Miccinati, Jeannette, "The Fernald technique: Modifications increase the probability of success," *Journal of Learning Disabilities* Vol. 12, No. 3 (March 1979), pp. 6–9.

Micklos, John, "Reading levels of newspapers," *Reading Today '84* Vol. 1, No. 4 (February 1984), International Reading Association.

Miles, T. R., *Dyslexia, the Pattern of Difficulties* (Springfield, Illinois: Charles C. Thomas, 1983).

Miles, T. R., and Miles, Elaine, *Help for Dyslexic Children* (London: Methuen, 1983).

Miller, George A. *The Psychology of Communication* (New York: Basic Books, 1967).

Money, John, ed., *Reading Disability, Progress and Research Needs in Dyslexia* (Baltimore: The Johns Hopkins Press, 1962).

Morency, Anne, "Auditory modality, research and practice," in Helen K. Smith, ed., *Perception and Reading* (Newark, Delaware: International Reading Association, 1968), Vol. 12, Part 4, pp. 17–21.

Morgan, W. Pringle, "A case of congenital word blindness," *British Medical Journal* (Nov. 7, 1896), p. 1378.

Mussen, Paul Henry, Conger, John Janeway, and Kagan, Jerome, *Readings in Child Development and Personality*, 2nd ed. (New York: Harper and Row, 1970).

Myklebust, Helmer J., *Development and Disorders of Written Language, Picture Story Language Test* Vol. 1 (New York: Grune and Stratton, 1965).

_____, *Development and Disorders of Written Language, Studies of Normal and Exceptional Children* Vol. 2 (New York: Grune and Stratton, 1973).

_____, ed., *Progress in Learning Disabilities* Vol. II (New York: Grune and Stratton, 1971).

_____, ed., *Progress in Learning Disabilities* Vol. IV (New York: Grune and Stratton, 1978).

Naidoo, Sandhya, *Specific Dyslexia, The Research Report of the ICAA Word Blind Centre for Dyslexic Children* (New York: John Wiley and Sons, 1972).

_____, "Symposium on reading disability: Specific developmental dyslexia," *British Journal of Educational Psychology* Vol. 41 (February 1971), pp. 19–21.

NATO Advanced Study Institute on Dyslexia: A Global Issue, Dyslexia, The Hague Boston published in cooperation with NATO Scientific Affairs Division (Hingham, MA: M. Nishoff, 1984).

Newton, Margaret, and Thomson, Michael, *Dyslexia, A Guide for Teachers and Parents* (London: University of London Press, 1975).

Noblitt, Gerald L., "Rejoinder on using scores from standardized reading tests," *The Reading Teacher* Vol. 36, No. 4 (January 1983), pp. 452–453.

Norrie, E., "Ordblindhedens (dyslexiens) arvegang. Laesepaedagogen" 2 (1954), p. 61 as cited in Knud Hermann *Reading Disability, A Medical Study of Word-Blindness and Related Handicaps* (Springfield, Illinois: Charles C. Thomas, 1959), and by Edith Zerbin-Rubin, "Congenital word-blindness," *Bulletin of the Orton Society* Vol. 17 (1967), pp. 45–55.

Olson, David R., "Language and thought: Aspects of a cognitive theory of semantics," *Psychological Review* 77 (July 1970), pp. 257–273.

Orton, Samuel T., " 'Word-blindness' in school children," *Archives of Neurology and Psychiatry* Vol. 14, No. 5 (November 1925), pp. 581–615.

_____, *Reading, Writing and Speech Problems in Children* (New York: W. W. Norton, 1937).

Otto, Wayne, and Smith, Richard J., *Corrective and Remedial Teaching* (Boston: Houghton Mifflin, 1980).

Owen, Freda W., Adams, P. A., Forrest, T., Stolz, L. M., and Fisher, S., "Learning disorders in children: Sibling studies," *Monographs of the Society for Research in Child Development* Vol. 36 (Chicago: University of Chicago, 1971).

Palermo, David S., and Molfese, Dennis L., "Language acquisition from age five onward," *Psychological Bulletin* Vol. 78, No. 6 (December 1972), pp. 409–428.

Pavlidis, George, and Mills, T.R., eds., *Dyslexia Research and Its Applications to Education* (New York: John Wiley and Sons, 1981).

Pearson, P. David, ed., *Reading: Theory, Research and Practice* (Clemson, South Carolina: The National Reading Conference, 1977).

Petty, Walter T., Petty, Dorothy C., and Becking, Marjorie F., *Experiences in Language, Tools and Techniques for Language Arts Methods* (Boston: Allyn and Bacon, 1973).

Petty, Walter T., and Jensen, Julie M., *Developing Children's Language* (Boston: Allyn and Bacon, 1980).

Piaget, Jean, "The stages of the intellectual development of the child," in Paul Henry Mussen, John Janeway Conger, and Jerome Kagan, eds., *Readings in Child Development and Personality*, 2nd ed. (New York: Harper and Row, 1970), pp. 291–298.

Picturesque Word Origins (Springfield, Mass.: G and C Merriam Company, 1933).

Public Law 94-142, Education of the Handicapped Act of 1975. The implementation of Part B dealing with specific learning disabilities, *Federal Register* (Dec. 29, 1977), effective September 1978.

Purtell, Thelma C., *Can't Read, Can't Write, Can't Takl Too Good Either* (New York: Walker, 1973).

Rawson, Margaret B., *Developmental Language Disability: Adult Accomplishments of Dyslexic Boys* (Baltimore: Johns Hopkins, 1968).

"Reading disorders in children," *The Journal of the American Medical Association* Vol. 206, No. 3 (Oct. 14, 1968).

"Readings . . . Finding New York's Finest," *Harper's* (February, 1986), pp. 16–18.

Reid, D. Kim, and Hresko, Wayne P., eds., *Topics in Learning and Learning Disabilities: Issues in Reading Diagnosis* Vol. 2, No. 4 (January 1983) (Gaithersburg, Pa: Aspen Systems).

Restak, Richard M., *The Brain* (New York: Bantam Books, 1984).

Ringler, Lenore H. and Weber, Carol K., *A Language-Thinking Approach to Reading Diagnosis and Teaching* (New York: Harcourt Brace Jovanovich, 1984).

Robeck, Mildred C., and Wilson, John A. R., *Psychology of Reading: Foundations of Instruction* (New York: John Wiley and Sons, 1974).

Rockefeller, Nelson A., "Don't accept anyone's verdict that you are lazy, stupid or retarded," *TV Guide* (Oct. 16, 1978), pp. 12–14.

"The Role of the Ophthalmologist in Dyslexia," Report of an international seminar held in Indianapolis, Indiana; Institute for Development of Educational Activities, an affiliate of the Charles F. Kettering Foundation, IDEA, Melbourne, Florida, 1969.

Rourke, Byron P., Bakker, Dirk J., Fisk, John L., and Strang, John D., *Child Neuropsychology, an Introduction to Theory, Research, and Clinical Practice* (New York: Guilford Press, 1983).

Rowe, Mary Budd, "Wait-time and rewards as instructional variables, their influence on language, logic, and fate control: Part one—wait-time," *Journal of Research in Science Teaching* Vol. 2 (1974), pp. 81–94.

Rowse, A. L., "Why a contemporary Shakespeare?" in *King Lear* (Lanham, Maryland: University Press of America, 1984), pp. 3–19.

Rupley, William H., and Blair, Timothy R., *Reading Diagnosis and Remediation* (Chicago, Illinois: Rand McNally, 1983).

Rutherford, "What is your D.Q. (Dyslexia Quotient)?" *The Reading Teacher* Vol. 25 (December 1971), pp. 262–266.

Samuels, S. Jay, "Diagnosing reading problems," *Topics in Learning and Learning Disabilities: Issues in Reading Diagnosis* Vol. 2, No. 4 (January 1983) (Gaithersburg, Pa.: Aspen Systems), pp. 1–11.

Satz, Paul, and Sparrow, Sara S., "Specific developmental dyslexia: A theoretical formulation," in Dirk J. Bakker and Paul Satz, eds., *Specific Reading Disability: Advances in Theory and Method* (The Netherlands: Rotterdam University Press, 1970), p. 17 ff.

Schiller, M., "Zwillingsprobleme, dargestellt auf Grund von Unter-suchungen an Stuttgarter Zwillingen," *Z. Menschl. Vererb.—U. Konstit.—Lehre* 20 (1937), p. 284, as cited in Edith Zerbin-Rubin, " Congenital word-blindness," *Bulletin of the Orton Society* Vol. 17 (1967), pp. 47–54.

Schmitt, Clara, "Developmental alexia: Congenital word-blindness or inability to learn to read," *The Elementary School Journal* Vol. 18 (1918), pp. 680–688.

School, Beverly A., and Cooper, Arlene, *The IEP Primer* (Novato, California: Academic Therapy, 1979).

Schwalb, Eugene, Blau, Harold, and Blau, Harriet, "Developmental and symptomatic Dyslexia: Differential diagnosis and remediation," in Barbara Bateman, ed., *Learning Disorders, Reading* Vol. 4 (1971) (Seattle, Washington: Special Child Publications), pp. 343–383.

Shuck, Annette, Ulsh, Florence, and Platt, John S., "Parents encourage pupils (PEP): An inner-city parent involvement reading project," *The Reading Teacher* Vol. 36, No. 6 (February 1983), pp. 524–528.

Silver, Archie A., and Hagin, Rosa A., "Specific reading disability: A twelve-year follow-up study," *American Journal of Ortho-psychiatry* Vol. 33 (March 1963), pp. 338–339.

_____. "Specific reading disability: Follow-up studies," *American Journal of Orthopsychiatry* Vol. 34, No. 1 (1964), pp. 95–102.

Sittig, Linda Harris, "Involving parents and children in reading for fun," *The Reading Teacher* Vol. 36, No. 2 (November, 1982), pp. 166–168.

Slobin, Dan I., *Psycholinguistics* (Glenview, Illinois: Scott, Foresman, 1971).

Smith, Frank, ed., *Psycholinguistics and Reading* (New York: Holt, Rinehart and Winston, 1973).

Smith, Frank, *Reading Without Nonsense* (New York: Teachers College, Columbia University, 1979).

_____, *Understanding Reading* (New York: Holt, Rinehart and Winston, 1971).

Smith, Frank, and Miller, George A., eds. *The Genesis of Language, A Psycholinguistic Approach* (Cambridge, Mass.: The M.I.T. Press, 1966).

Smith, Lawrence L., Johns, Jerry L., Ganschow, Leonore, and Masztal, Nancy Browning, "Using grade level vs. out-of-level reading tests with remedial students," *The Reading Teacher* Vol. 36, No. 6 (February 1983), pp. 550–553.

Smith, Nancy J., "The word processing approach to language ex-perience," *The Reading Teacher* Vol. 38 (February 1985), pp. 556–559.

Smith, R. J. and Johnson, D. D., *Teaching Children to Read*, 2nd ed. (Reading, Mass.: Addison-Wesley, 1980).

Smith, Shelley D., Kimberling, William J., Pennington, Bruce F., and Lubs, Herbert A., "Specific reading disability: Identification of an inherited form through linkage analysis," *Science* Vol. 219, (March 18, 1983), pp. 1345–1347.

Snow, Katherine, "A comparative study of sound substitutions used by 'normal' first grade children," *Speech Monographs* 31 (1964), pp. 135–142.

Spache, George D., *Diagnosing and Correcting Reading Disabilities*, 2nd ed. (Boston: Allyn and Bacon, 1981).

Sperling, George, "Short-term memory, long-term memory, and scanning in the processing of visual information," in Francis A. Young and Donald B. Lindsley, eds., *Early Experience and Visual Information Processing in Perceptual and Reading Disorders* (Washington, D.C.: National Academy of Sciences, 1970), pp. 198–215.

Spiel, W., "Beitrag zur kongenitalen Lese—und Schreibstörung," *Wien Z. Nervenheilk* 7 (1953), p. 20, as cited in Edith Zerbin-Rubin "Congenital word-blindness," *Bulletin of the Orton Society* Vol. 17 (1967), pp. 47–54.

Stauffer, Russell, Abrams, Jules C., and Pikulski, John J., *Diagnosis, Correction, and Prevention of Reading Disabilities* (New York: Harper and Row, 1978).

Stevenson, Lillian P., "WISC-R analysis: Implications for diagnosis and intervention," *Journal of Learning Disabilities* Vol. 13, No. 6 (June/July 1980), pp. 60–63.

Strauss, Alfred A., and Lehtinen, Laura E., *Psychopathology and Education of the Brain-Injured Child* (New York: Grune and Stratton, 1947).

Taylor, Pamela, *The Notebooks of Leonardo da Vinci*. (New York: New American Library, 1960).

Taylor, Robert Lewis, *Winston Churchill, An Informal Study of Greatness* (Garden City, New York: Doubleday, 1952).

Taylor, Stanford E., "Listening," *What Research Says to the Teacher* No. 29 (1964) (Washington, D.C.: National Education Association).

Temple, Charles, and Gillet, Jean Wallace, *Language Arts, Learning Processes and Teaching Practices* (Boston: Little, Brown, 1984).

Templeton, Shane, "Spelling, phonology and the older student," in Edmund H. Henderson and James W. Beers, eds., *Developmental and Cognitive Aspects of Learning to Spell: A Reflection of Word Knowledge* (Newark, Delaware: International Reading Association, 1980), pp. 85–96.

Templin, Mildred C., "The study of articulation and language development during the early school years," *A Genesis of Language, A Psycholinguistic Approach* (Cambridge, Mass.: The M.I.T. Press, 1966), pp. 173–180.

Thomas, James Blake, *Introduction to Human Embryology* (Philadelphia. Lea and Febiger, 1968)

Thompson, Lloyd J., "Language disabilities in men of eminence," *Journal of Learning Disabilities* Vol. 4 (January 1971), pp. 34–45.

Thomson, Michael, *Developmental Dyslexia* (London: Edward Arnold Publishers Ltd., 1984).

Tomkins, Calvin, "The last skill acquired," *New Yorker* 39 (Sept. 14, 1963), pp. 127–157.

Turaids, Dainis, Wepman, Joseph M., and Morency, Anne, "A perceptual test battery: Development and standardization," *Elementary School Journal* Vol. 72, No. 7 (April 1972), pp. 351–361.

Valett, Robert E., *Dyslexia, a Neuropsychological Approach to Educating Children With Severe Reading Disorders* (Belmont, California: Fearon Pitman, 1980).

Varney, Nils R., and Damasio, Antonio R., "Acquired dyslexia," in R. N. Malatesha and P. G. Aaron, eds., *Reading Disorders, Varieties and Treatments* (New York: Academic Press, 1982), pp. 305–314.

Vawter, Jacquelyn M., and Vancil, Marybelle, "Helping children discover reading through self-directed dramatization," *The Reading Teacher* Vol. 34, No. 3 (December 1980), pp. 320–323.

Veatch, Florence Sawicki, Elliott, Geraldine, Barnette, Eleanor, and Blakey, Janis, *Key Words to Reading: The Language Approach Begins* (Columbus, Ohio: Charles E. Merrill, 1973).

Vellutino, Frank, "Dyslexia: Perceptual deficiency or perceptual inefficiency," in James F. Kavanagh and Richard L. Venezky, eds., *Orthography, Reading, and Dyslexia* (Baltimore: University Park Press, 1980), pp. 251–270.

_____, *Dyslexia: Theory and Research* (Cambridge: The M.I.T. Press, 1979).

Venezky, Richard L., "Regularity in reading and spelling," in Harry Levin and Joanna P. Williams, eds., *Basic Studies on Reading* (New York: Basic Books, 1970), pp. 30–42.

Vernon, M. D., *Backwardness in Reading, A Study of its Nature and Origin* (Cambridge: Cambridge University Press, 1958).

Vogel, Susan Ann, *Syntactic Abilities in Normal and Dyslexic Children* (Baltimore: University Park Press, 1975).

vonHarnack, (1948) as cited in Edith Zerbin-Rubin, "Congenital word-blindness," *Bulletin of the Orton Society* Vol. 17 (1967), pp. 47–54.

Vukelich, Carol, "Parents' role in the reading process: A review of practical suggestions and ways to communicate with parents," *The Reading Teacher* Vol. 37, No. 6 (February 1984), pp. 472–477.

Wagner, Rudolph F., *Dyslexia and Your Child* (New York: Harper and Row, 1971).

_____, "Rudolph Berlin: Originator of the term dyslexia," *Bulletin of the Orton Society* Vol. 23 (1973), pp. 57–63.

Wallace, Gerald, and McLoughlin, James A., *Learning Disabilities, Concepts and Characteristics* (Columbus, Ohio: Charles E. Merrill, 1975).

Waller, T. Gary, and MacKinnon, G. E., eds., *Reading Research, Advances in Theory and Practice* (New York: Academic Press, 1979).

Wardhaugh, Ronald, *Reading: A Linguistic Perspective* (New York: Harcourt, Brace and World, 1969).

Weinschenk, C., "Die erbliche Lese-Rechtschreibeschwache and ihre sozialpsychiatrischen Auswirkungen," Schweiz. *Z. Psychol. Beih* (1962), p. 44 as cited in Edith Zerbin-Rubin, "Congenital word-blindness," *Bulletin of the Orton Society* Vol. 17 (1967), pp. 47–54.

Welchman, and Will, Stewart Obe, "Dyslexia 1972–1982," *British Dyslexia Association* (Peppard, Oxfordshire: British Dyslexia Association, 1982).

Wheeler, T. J., and Watkins, E. J., "Dyslexia: A review of symptomatology," *Dyslexia Review* 2, No. 1 (1979), pp. 12–16.

Wiegel-Crump, Carole Ann, "Rehabilitation of acquired dyslexia of adolescence," in T. Gary Waller and G. E. Mackinnon, eds., *Reading Research, Advances in Theory and Practice* Vol. 1 (New York: Academic Press, 1979), pp. 171–186.

Wildman, Terry M., "Cognitive theory and the design of instruction," *Educational Technology* (July 1981), pp. 14–19.

Wilson, Edith Bolling, *My Memoir* (New York: Bobbs-Merrill 1938).

Wilson, Louis Ada, "A study of some influencing factors upon and the nature of young children's written language," *The Journal of Experimental Education* Vol. 31, No. 4 (Summer 1963), pp. 371–380.

Wilson, Robert M., *Diagnostic and Remedial Reading for Classroom and Clinic*, 4th ed. (Columbus, Ohio: Charles E. Merrill, 1981).

Young, Francis A., and Lindsley, Donald B., eds., *Early Experience and Visual Information Processing in Perceptual and Reading Disorders* (Washington, D.C.: National Academy of Sciences, 1970).

Zerbin-Rubin, Edith, "Congenital word-blindness," *Bulletin of the Orton Society* Vol. 17 (1967), pp. 47–55.

Zintz, Miles V., *Corrective Reading* (Dubuque, Iowa: Wm. C. Brown, 1981).

Zintz, Miles V., and Maggart, Zelda R., *The Reading Process, the Teacher and the Learner*, 4th ed. (Dubuque, Iowa: Wm. C. Brown, 1984).

INDEX

Barnett, Lincoln, 22
Bateman, Barbara, 39
BEAM. See brain electrical
  activity mapping
Beers, James W. 22, 84–85
Bender, Michael, 139
Bender Visual-Motor Gestalt
  test, 78, 81, 85
Benton, Arthur L., 85, 86, 124
Berlin, Rudolph, 99, 100
birth order of dyslexics, 9
Blackburn, J., 38, 124
Blair, Timothy R., 84
blueprints. See floor plans
boarding schools, 204–205
Boder, Elena, 38–39
book clubs, 189
books
  high-interest, low vocabulary,
    178–179
  rewriting, 210–211
  subject matter, 211
Boyd, Gertrude A., 85
brain
  angular gyrus, 98, 101
  auditory region, 121
  Broca's area, 117
  central fissure, 103
  cerebral damage, 102
  cognitive strategies, 116
  cortex, 103, 120, 121
  electrical activity mapping
    (BEAM), 114–115
  hemispheres, 103, 110, 111,
    116–118, 119, 120, 213
  of a dyslexic, 119–121
  language areas, 120, 124
  mirror images, 102, 111–112,
    116
  myelination, brain cells,
    81–82, 120
  occipital lobe, 103
  parietal lobe, 103

planum temporale, 121
Broadbent, Sir William H., 98,
  99, 102
Broman, Betty L., 85
Buckley Amendment, 203–204
Burg, Leslie, 225
Burns, Paul C., 85

C

calculator, 143, 189
Calder, Richie, 161, 170
Caldarelli, David D., 69
Campanella, Ruth S., 69
career choices, 143, 145–146
case studies, five children, 87–96
causes of dyslexia, theories,
  105–125
  cerebellar-vestibular (C–V)
    dysfunction, 121–123
  cerebral dominance, 110–112
  congenital, 101
  genetic, 106–109
  maturational lag, 109–110
  neurological dysfunction,
    112–113
  specialization within brain,
    116–119
central nervous system, 110, 112
cerebral immaturity, 109, 110
Charles XI, King, 154, 155–156
Childs, Anne L., 124
Childs, Barton, 124, 149
Churchill, Sir Winston, 154,
  155–158
chunking, 31–32
Clouse, Robert G., 171
classroom environment,
  209–210
coding, 54, 68, 143, 159
cognitive development, 75,
  80–81

categories, 5, 26
common characteristics of
categories, 26–34
definition, 5
diagnosis, 25–26, 152
early identification, 73–86
five children, 87–96
based on spelling errors,
38–39, 164, 168
pseudodyslexic symptoms,
42–44, 61–63, 152
genetic causes, 106–109
historical development of
concept, 97–103
incidence of, 6–7
information processing, 12
meaning, critical element,
31–32
middle school and high
school, 129–139
percentage of cases, 6–7, 26
socioeconomic background, 9
subtypes, 5, 26
teacher training, 218–219

E

ear, main parts of, 59–61
early identification of dyslexia,
73–86, 109, 219
Edison, Thomas, 154, 155–159
Educational Testing Service
(ETS), 138
Edwards, R. Philip, 85
electroencephalogram (EEG),
113–114, 219
critique of studies, 124
Ehrlich, Paul, 167
Einstein, Albert, 8–9, 154,
159–161
Ekwall, Eldon E., 84
Elkind, David, 124
environment, 186–187

sensitivity to noise and
movement, 30
examinations, 212
experience charts, 90, 91, 179,
221
extra-personal space awareness,
79
eye-hand coordination, 77–79
eye movements, 15, 16

F

Family Education Rights and
Privacy Act, (FERPA), 203–204
family history studies, 106–109
family mailbox, 191
family relationships, 146–148
Farago, Ladislas, 170
farsighted, 74
Fernald, Grace, 170
films, 211–212
finger agnosia, 37, 81, 120,
152, 154
Finucci, Joan M., 124, 149
Fisk, John L., 124
Fleming, Elizabeth, 171
floor plans, 55
fluency, 32
foreign language, 68, 131, 153,
165
movie subtitles, 143
requirements eliminated, 131
Francone, Clarice Ashworth,
58, 69
Frauenheim, John G., 139
free reading level, 27, 188
Funk, Hal D., 22

G

Galaburda, Albert M., 119–121,
124